WOMEN
AND
STRESS

D0951788

Another book by Jean Lush with Pam Vredevelt
Mothers and Sons: Raising Boys to Be Men

Other books by Pam Vredevelt
Angel Behind the Rocking Chair: Stories of Hope in Unexpected Places

Empty Arms: Hope and Support for Those Who Have Suffered a Miscarriage, Stillbirth, or Tubal Pregnancy

Espresso for a Woman's Spirit: Encouraging Stories of Hope and Humor (Espresso)

Espresso for a Woman's Spirit 2: More Encouraging Stories of Hope and Humor (Espresso)

Espresso for Your Spirit: Hope and Humor for Pooped-Out Parents (Espresso)

The Power of Letting Go: 10 Simple Steps to Reclaiming Your Life

The Thin Disguise: Understanding and Overcoming Anorexia & Bulimia (with Deborah Newman, Harry Beverly, and Frank Minirth)

The Wounded Woman: Hope and Healing for Those Who Hurt (with Steve Stephens)

WOMEN
AND
STRESS

PRACTICAL WAYS
to
MANAGE TENSION

JEAN LUSH
with PAM VREDEVELT

SPIRE

© 1992 by Jean Lush and Pam Vredevelt

"A Word from Pam" © 2008 by Pam Vredevelt

Published by Revell
a division of Baker Publishing Group
P.O. Box 6287, Grand Rapids, MI 49516-6287
www.revellbooks.com

Spire edition published 2011
ISBN 978-0-8007-8810-0

Previously published in 2008

Printed in the United States of America

All rights reserved. No part of this publication may be reproduced, stored in a re-
trieval system, or transmitted in any form or by any means—for example, electronic,
photocopy, recording—without the prior written permission of the publisher. The
only exception is brief quotations in printed reviews.

Unless otherwise indicated, Scripture is taken from the Holy Bible, New International
Version®. NIV®. Copyright © 1973, 1978, 1984, by Biblica, Inc.™ Used by permission
of Zondervan. All rights reserved worldwide. www.zondervan.com

Scripture marked AMP is taken from the Amplified© Bible, Copyright © 1954, 1958,
1962, 1964, 1965, 1987 by The Lockman Foundation. Used by permission.

Scripture marked TLB is taken from *The Living Bible*, copyright © 1971. Used by permission of Tyndale House Publishers, Inc., Wheaton, Illinois 60189. All rights reserved.

Material from the book *Empty Arms: Emotional Support for Those Who Have Suffered Miscarriage or Stillbirth* by Pam Vredevelt, copyright © 1984 by Multnomah
Press. Published by Multnomah Press, Portland, Oregon, 97266. Used by permission.

12 13 14 15 16 17 18   8 7 6 5 4 3

This book is dedicated to the memory of my husband, who always pushed me to discover a potential I never knew was there.

Contents

Contents

Introduction

If we were professors and you, the reader, were our student, this is what we would say to you about this book: This book is not an academic textbook on the subject of tension and stress. It is a compilation of practical ideas and vignettes that illustrate how women in today's world can rise above their tensions. You will meet real people with real struggles similar to your own. You will see the creative ways they tamed their tensions. After you have read this book, we think you will conclude, "If they can do it, so can I."

Jean Lush
Pam Vredevelt
1992

A Word from Pam

My first copy of *Women and Stress* arrived in the mail a few weeks after the traumatic birth of our son Nathan. Much to our astonishment, Nathan arrived six weeks early, with a surprise diagnosis of Down Syndrome and severe heart complications. As I flipped through my first copy of the book Jean Lush and I had poured our hearts into writing, I thought, "God knew I would need this book to survive this season of my life."

During the three years following Nathan's arrival, I read and re-read many of the chapters in *Women and Stress*. Jean's wisdom and colorful stories comforted me during a time when I was flooded with grief and overwhelmed by the demands of life. Her wisdom from the Lord—and from being a family therapist for over thirty years—empowered me to persevere and to make wise choices, especially during those times when I silently wondered if I could face one more day.

As the years have passed, I have had the privilege of sharing the timeless truths in *Women and Stress* with thousands of women. In the counseling office, I witness women experiencing breakthroughs and newfound freedom as they apply these principles to their lives. When I travel and speak at women's events across the nation, it is the same everywhere: women are stressed, and are looking for practical ways to manage their tension, balance their lives, and experience more peace.

I'm forever grateful for the privilege of writing two books with Jean. She was one of the most intelligent, intuitive, and humble women I've ever met. Her sixth sense into human nature never ceased to amaze me. Younger generations may not be aware that Jean was one of Dr. James Dobson's most frequent and popular talk show guests on "Focus on the Family". I believe she did her first radio show with him when she was in her seventies. Jean is now with the Lord in heaven, free from the stress of this world.

When my time on earth is finished, I imagine she will greet me with open arms, invite me over for a cup of her famous English tea, and, in keeping with her style, say: "Welcome home, Ducky! It's time for a real good rest. The Lord knows you deserve it!"

Pam Vredevelt

WHAT MAKES
US TENSE?

1

Anger

My good friend Rachael and I had invited missionary Jill Torrey-Renich to speak at our three-day evangelistic rally in Australia. Jill and her husband had been involved in great revival ministries in Ireland and England; she had also been a missionary in China. A descendant of the great R. A. Torrey, Jill had spiritual genes, and we knew she would have a tremendous impact on our women. I never anticipated a personal prophetic warning.

I remember Jill's words as if they were spoken yesterday: "It will be a long time before I see you two again, and I have a prophetic message for you. In all my traveling years I have never seen anything like this group. You girls have a very effective ministry, and the devil is bound to strike. I have strong feelings that he will aim his darts at your relationship. If he breaks your unity as leaders, he can destroy the group."

At the time her warning seemed ridiculous. I almost burst out laughing. After all, Rachael and I had had our babies together. We were soul mates who shared everything—our joys, our sorrows, even our vacations.

"Australians don't go for that kind of talk," I said to Jill. "Maybe on your missionary journeys you're used to thinking about that devil stuff, but Australians don't mess with it. When problems come, we see ourselves as the cause, take the conflicts in stride, and plunge ahead."

After the weekend crusade, I traveled back to my family in the beautiful hills outside the city of Adelaide. Three acres of gardens and walnut orchards set among giant eucalyptus trees kept me very busy, as did my three grade-school children. When I wasn't supervising the kids, there were chickens, several pets, and our huge black-and-white cow to keep me on the run.

I thanked God for our women's fellowship group. It was a great outlet from the pressures of life. That year there was a great polio epidemic in the city. Over two thousand people, mostly children, died of the disease. We carefully kept our children at home to avoid exposure. For months they didn't have the pleasure of playing with children from other families. My husband, Lyall, was frequently absent because of his occupation and ministry. This left me with an incredible burden to bear on my own.

World War II also affected us. Japanese submarines were in the bay, and Australia was on a wartime footing. Cars and telephones were scarce; civilians were allowed one telephone per block of homes, and families were restricted to three gallons of gasoline a month. This made traveling to the city from our home in the hills next to impossible. We had to save our gasoline strictly for emergency purposes.

Two to three months after Jill Torrey spoke at our crusade, a neighbor from several blocks away came running to my house with an urgent telephone message from Rachael.

Much to my surprise, she said Rachael was on her way up the mountain to talk to me. I couldn't imagine what would prompt her to waste so much gas.

When I heard her car pull up to the house, I dashed out to see what was the matter. Storming toward the front door, she blurted out, "Jean, I must talk to you alone. My news isn't pleasant, but you simply must know what everyone is saying about Lyall!"

"What are you talking about, Rachael?" I said in amazement.

Rachael spoke straight to the point. "Jean, as your friend, I felt I must tell you what I heard in my house over tea. Lyall is the center of everyone's discussions. Do you realize that Lyall's business is in a dreadful mess? People are saying he is cheating his employees. Apparently he is consistently losing his clients. Lyall goes off and preaches for days at a time, irresponsibly leaving the business to his employees. People don't think Lyall should be involved in ministry if he is going to carry on with shabby business practices."

Rachael left suddenly. I sat in my parlor, stunned by what had just happened. My mind replayed her words again and again. In moments I was demented by anger. How dare my best friend be a party to this gossip in her home? Rachael's house was in the middle of the city and served as a meeting place for many of the women in our fellowship group. Not once had she mentioned these rumors during the weeks they had been swapped across her kitchen table! I was outraged by her betrayal.

I knew without a doubt that Lyall was a man of impeccable honor and integrity. There were times when I felt he was almost too conscientious and responsible. His deep devotion to God and strict professionalism made me confident that Rachael's information was terribly wrong.

Rachael's message came on a Friday. After tucking the children into bed, I tried to sleep but lay awake into the early morning hours, obsessed with anger. On Saturday I was useless and couldn't function around the house. My mind refused to concentrate on anything except devising a plan for revenge. I had never experienced such murderous feelings that screamed for action. I desperately wanted to hurt Rachael. She had to be punished.

Perhaps you're asking, "Why didn't you calmly investigate and gather more information before becoming so enraged?"

Believe me, I would have loved to have had more information, but I was stuck. I had no way to uncover the facts. My husband was out of town, I had no telephone, and we didn't have the funds for a long-distance call on the telephone down the street.

My emotions ran wild and unchecked. I simply was not able to say to myself: "Hey, you silly person, don't feel angry. You know there's more to the story than you've heard. Keep calm until you find out more information."

A high level of tension does that to us. It throws off our equilibrium. Neon *tilt* lights flash; our wires short-circuit; sparks fly; smoke billows. All functions grind to a halt.

Our wiring actually does get maxed-out when we are under prolonged periods of stress. "Too Much Stress Burns Out Brain Cells" is the title of an article that discusses recent research finds. Whenever a person moves into a flight-or-fight response to stressful situations, adrenaline and cortisol are released into the bloodstream by the adrenal glands. Apparently, prolonged exposure to stress and the continual release of these hormones can accelerate the aging of brain cells and lead to the impairment of learning and memory.[1]

Tension and stress—I see them as one in the same. Webster's Dictionary says that stress is a condition in which an individual fails to make a satisfactory adaptation. It's synonymous with *strain*, *pressure*, and *tension*.[2] The Latin root of the word *stress* is "strengere," meaning to bind tight.[3] There are many definitions of *stress*, but I like one used by heart researcher Dr. Redford Williams best. He says stress is any bit of sensory information that makes its way to the brain and changes the brain's communication to the body.[4]

Tension can be caused by a number of sources. Anything that annoys, threatens, prods, excites, scares, worries, hurries, angers, frustrates, challenges, criticizes, or reduces our self-esteem will cause tension. Stress-management expert Dr. Hans Selye says that anything that challenges the body's equilibrium and puts it into an emergency mode will cause stress damage over time.[5]

During the last twenty years, when I've taught audiences about taming their tensions, I've used a simple diagram that shows what happens to us when we are feeling tense.

We start with a negative stimulus, anything that upsets us. Any time we are confronted with a negative stimulus, we feel tension. Tension is energy. When we are frustrated or angry in response to a negative stimulus, high levels of energy swirl around inside us. Our emotions are aroused.

Now this next point is important: Tension is energy, and energy will always strive to be discharged, so when we are tense, we are carrying high levels of emotional energy constantly striving to be discharged. Discharge comes in a variety of ways, depending on how we manage our "storage pots."

Some people have pots with a very small storage capacity. They rarely close the lids. I call these people Fighters. Whenever they are tense, they immediately unload their tension, regardless of the cost. They act out their emotions.

Other people have a very large storage capacity; they rarely open the lids on their pots. I call these people Flighters. Since the tension isn't discharged outwardly, it gets discharged inwardly. Flighters commonly suffer psychosomatic illnesses, depression, avoidance, and procrastination.

My immediate response to Rachael's sudden negative stimulus was anger. High levels of tension were striving for discharge—I wanted revenge. My Christian upbringing created further conflict. I heard part of me saying: "Jean, these awful feelings must be classified as ego alien to you. Especially to you, since you are in Christian service." I know anger isn't unspiritual, but at the time, these were the thoughts dashing through my mind.

Sunday morning I told the children, "You are going to church and Christian Endeavor meeting, as well as Sunday school this afternoon. I am staying home." They grumbled that I wasn't being fair, but I sent them on their way.

Alone in the quiet of my home, I felt a war raging in my heart. My plan for revenge energized me with a sense of power, but my intense desire to destroy my best friend frightened me. I had never experienced such hostile impulses in all my life.

Then it happened. Walking through the house, I was stopped cold in my tracks when the prophetic warning from Jill Torrey flashed through my mind: "Jean and Rachael, the devil will strike at your friendship. Be on guard. The enemy will try to tear you two apart, and this will destroy your women's fellowship."

God was speaking to me. I wanted to hear more. Opening my Bible, I prepared to listen. The Lord began to instruct me from Psalm 37, underlining truths He specifically wanted me to grasp.

"Trust in Me."

"I will grant your heart's desires."

"Trust in Me."

"I will act."

"Wait quietly for Me . . . be patient."

"Be angry no more."

"Don't strive to do evil."

"I am holding you by the hand."

"Turn from evil and do good."

"Wait."

The Holy Spirit kept bringing me back to those poignant but very difficult words, "Wait quietly."

"But God, this is an impossible assignment. Everything in me is craving retribution. I don't know if I can hold myself together. I feel compelled to act!"

Then came His promise: "I am holding you by the hand."

If I would do my part, He would do His. If I chose to obey Him, He would enable me to sit tight.

I was left with a choice. Would I move on my hostile impulses to get even with Rachael, or would I obey God and wait quietly while He took care of the problem?

I knelt down beside my grandmother's old Victorian chair and prayed. "Oh, God, I will obey You. I will not strike out and hurt Rachael. But please, God, help me. I cannot get rid of my anger. I can't make these awful feelings go away." My prayer was not a passive reaction to my problem. I aggressively chose to contain my impulses to act.

Rising from my knees, I felt the anger continue, but the hostility was not as all-consuming as before. The quiet Sunday morning was nearly gone, and I had a dinner to prepare for my family, who would soon bound through the door. Walking to the kitchen, I sensed I was different—some of the heaviness had lifted, and I had the energy to concentrate on the household again.

Monday morning dawned, and all the horrors of wash day were upon me: heating up the water in the big copper boiler, stoking the fire under the washtub, wringing garments through the old hand wringer, carrying the heavy basket of wet clothes up the slope to the clothesline in 100-degree heat, hoping for a gust of wind to cool me, scrubbing out the washhouse, mopping down the large kitchen floor, and cleaning out the ashes. I don't think I had the energy to give Rachael much thought that day.

Tuesday came and went without any major upheavals. Every now and then, when I thought of Rachael, anger surfaced, but I was no longer immobilized by the situation.

Then came another message from a neighbor. She said I must run immediately to the phone up the hill to take an urgent call.

I had barely said hello when Rachael's words tumbled out. "Oh, Jean, can you ever forgive me? When I got home Friday night, Mark was furious with me for taking the car and wasting our gas. When I told him why I had gone to your home, he said I had made a fool of myself and that we were going to be the laughingstock of all our business friends. He said the rumors were started by a person in Lyall's company who wanted to discredit Lyall to steal his business. Mark accused me of being a treacherously vicious gossip. He ordered me to call you and apologize. Oh, Jean, I feel simply awful!"

As I listened to her frantic voice, I felt so sorry for her. "Rachael, of course I forgive you. Let's put this nonsense behind us forever. We don't need to talk about it again. Let's get on with our vision."

To my surprise, I meant every word. God had been faithful to help me let go of my anger. Offering Rachael forgiveness had nothing to do with her apology and everything to do with my choice to trust Him to work things out His way. Forgiveness wasn't a gift I gave Rachael; it was a gift I gave myself. It opened the door of my soul and booted out my hostilities.

But suppose Rachael had not apologized? There have been those in my life who haven't. What if there had been no quick resolution to the conflict? What if the walls between us had become larger with time? The chapters that follow will address several inescapable sources of tension. Read on and discover what you can do when it's impossible to make your source of tension disappear.

2

Painful Emotions

There are certain painful emotions that will always cause us to suffer tension until we root them out of our lives. Among the most powerful of these are guilt, fear, envy, and jealousy. Until we learn to control these emotions, we will suffer from incredible tension.

Guilt

"I just don't understand! Michael has always been easygoing, but lately he's a bundle of nerves. He snaps at me and the kids over nothing. Yesterday our four-year-old left his tricycle out in the rain, and Michael exploded. I've never seen him that mad. His face turned beet red, and he screamed so loud that the whole neighborhood heard him." With a look of despair, she threw up her hands, saying, "I don't know what to do!"

Margaret was a busy young wife and mother of three children. For eight years she and Michael had been happily married, but something had changed in the last six months, and she was concerned. Michael was distant and irritable, and she wanted to know what she could do to help.

I asked about his job, knowing this is a chief source of strain for most men. She told me he had received glowing evaluations and a pay raise in the last year. Weeks later I called Michael and asked him to meet with me alone, to help me better understand his wife. I requested one hour of his time, hoping I could form a better picture of what was going on. To my surprise, he agreed to the meeting.

The picture began to unfold. Michael was a devoted family man, but he was attracted to his bright young secretary. Their lunches together had started out as harmless fun, but now he was overly attracted to her. He fantasized about the great team they would make in the workplace. He knew they could climb the corporate ladder together and be a smashing success.

Michael was an ambitious young man, but he lacked self-confidence. His secretary met this need by taking a genuine interest in his future and dedicating herself to his cause. You can imagine the fantasies that were flying around in her mind, too.

Conflict was also brewing in his marriage. Michael wanted Margaret to take more interest in the firm, but she wanted him to forget work when he was home and concentrate on the family. When he was home, he wanted to be back at the office. Longings for his secretary increased, and so did his guilt. Soon he dreaded going to church and made excuses to stay home. "I'm just too tired," was the standard reason given.

By now you may be saying, "I don't get it. Michael is the one who is messing around on his wife, so why is he giving her and the kids a bad time? They haven't done anything."

That's how we act when we feel guilty. We cast our ugly feelings onto others. Michael's guilt over his double life drove him to dump his anger-induced tension on Margaret and the children. Tension will always be discharged, and we rarely control that discharge wisely. Michael's guilt drove him to neurotic behavior that undermined his good judgment in business. Then sin became a stressor for him, as well.[1]

We experience peace when we live in a way that supports our values and beliefs. But when we go against our values, guilt causes us to feel angry, and we project our anger onto those around us. As S. I. McMillen says: "A clear conscience is a great step toward barricading the mind against neuroticism."[2]

However, I must include a word of caution here. I have heard of many cases where an unfaithful spouse felt it was necessary to be completely honest with his or her spouse in order to regain a clear conscience, and the mate never recovered from hearing the details. I believe there are times when other virtues must be placed higher than complete honesty. Sometimes honesty is a selfish effort to get rid of a burden of guilt. If we confess our wrongs to the Lord and to another and ask for forgiveness, that should often be the end of it. There are times when complete honesty is destructive to others we love and we cannot afford the luxury of "baring all" at the expense of someone else's well-being.

Michael knew Margaret would never be able to live with the truth. I sensed he was right. Michael was genuinely a family man, but he was also very ambitious. In counseling he began to see how he was using his secretary to get ahead. His attachment to her was very self-centered in nature. Confessing this to his wife might have relieved his conscience, but it would have destroyed Margaret and his marriage.

Michael's struggles are not uncommon. Men may want to be monogamous, but they find it difficult. When a man becomes a Christian, one of the biggest commitments he makes is to be faithful to his wife, but this is not easy for a man. Many Christian husbands tell me, "I hate being attracted to the good-looking women at work. When will I be free of this? I love my wife, and I don't want to have these feelings."

"I cannot answer your question," I respond, "but I will instruct you to *never* act on what you are feeling. You may not be able to get rid of your feelings, but you can control what you do with them. Make a firm commitment to be faithful to your wife. This will make a difference in the way you react to your feelings. Sometimes you will need to choose to act in ways that are totally contradictory to your feelings in order to protect your marriage."

Michael found this advice helpful. In time, he realized his anger was being caused by guilt and severed his romantic ties with his secretary. Changes at the office led to changes at home. As the guilt subsided, so did the anger and tension. Margaret didn't know about his involvement with his secretary; she only knew he was easier to live with, and figured he was coping better with business. Mercy took priority over honesty. Twenty years later, their marriage continues, and they are very much in love with each other.

Fear

Fear is another stressor that may cause us to lash out inappropriately in an attempt to reduce the tension tearing us apart.

Many years ago, a family doctor referred a fifty-five-year-old couple to me because the wife was experiencing symptoms he could not diagnose. After the husband's early retirement, they sold their old home and resettled in a small country town. The doctor wondered if the wife's symptoms were due to marital conflicts or some kind of adjustment problem.

I saw the wife alone, and she described varied and shifting symptoms. She complained, "Robert talks terribly mean to me whenever I'm ill. He treats me like I've done something bad. I need sympathy, not rage!"

Next I met with Robert. He came into my office obviously upset about his wife's illness. During our session I asked him why he was angry with his wife when she wasn't feeling well. His response was informative.

"Ma'am, I am so scared! My wife is all I have. We never had any kids. I know I say mean things to her, but I can't help it. I'm so afraid the doctors don't know what ails her. I know she's really sick, and they don't know how to make her well."

This dear man had every reason to be afraid. His premonition that his wife's condition was fatal was correct. One-and-a-half years later, she died of a brain tumor. Do you see how this husband vented his genuine fears through anger? It's unfortunate that the person he so dearly loved caught the brunt of his rage, but I know this isn't an isolated case. I've seen these dynamics played out in multitudes of homes.

As parents, we often discharge our fears through anger. What mother of preschoolers hasn't experienced this? I recall one young mother who taught her three-year-old boy to hold her hand whenever they took walks. On one occasion, they were strolling along a paved footpath next to a busy highway. Suddenly the little boy saw a tiny kitten mewing with terror on the other side of the road. He yanked his hand away and rushed into the road. The mother wasn't quick enough to grab him. Terrible fear knocked her to her knees. Two cars careened all over the road, trying to avoid the child. Next came the crunching noises of colliding cars.

The mother slapped her hands over her eyes, absolutely paralyzed. She knew her son could not make it across the road without being killed.

"I got the kitty, Mommy" were the next sounds she heard.

In a flash the little boy's mother was in the middle of the road, screaming at her son. "You naughty boy! You know better! Don't ever do that again as long as you live! You scared me to death!"

All the way home, she relived those horrifying moments, venting her anger on him. With every flashback came another surge of anger.

Oh, how many times I blew up at my children as a result of fear. If I could, I would go back and do things differently. I'd explain my fears to them and try to help them understand why I was angry. I don't have a second chance to raise my children, but I can use what I've learned with my grandchildren. When I'm afraid, they hear me say, "I may sound angry, but really I'm scared for you." This wins their ear much more effectively than a long-winded tirade.

Envy and Jealousy

Few things in life have the power jealousy and envy have to create volatile surges of tension in us. The energy stirred up by these emotions viciously strives toward discharge, often compelling people to do stupid things to find relief. Just look at the front page of your local newspaper, and you'll find plenty of examples. MAN SHOOTS WIFE. BROTHER

Murders Sister for Inheritance. The columns are filled with stories of people who senselessly act out their emotions.

The Old Testament contains plenty of stories of violence and jealousy. Think of Joseph, whose jealous brothers sold him into slavery. Then there was King Saul, who tried for years to murder David because of David's growing popularity among the subjects of Saul's kingdom.

The intense emotional pain created by jealousy and envy can drive people crazy, making them act in ways that are totally out of character. How often I have heard it said, "Harry was such a nice, quiet person. He never did anything to hurt anyone. I can't believe he killed his wife over her innocent friendship with her boss."

I've seen families split up because of jealousy and envy. One young man refused to speak to his four brothers and sisters after the reading of his parents' will. He felt the distribution of assets had been unfair and bitterly resented his siblings for getting certain parts of the estate that he thought were promised to him.

Many of the paranoid patients I treated suffered severe feelings of jealousy without reason. I could always tell when jealousy governed their relationships. They were ambivalent about their partners, unable to love, but desperately needed the feeling of being "in love."[3,4]

During my years of clinical work, I recall two great psychiatry professors saying that paranoid, jealous people need regular opportunities to vent their hurts and resentments. They should consistently be given a hearing, so they can let off steam and discharge their aggressive feelings.[5] Those who are permitted to talk openly about their conflicts on a weekly basis cope better with life and can restrain their impulses to lash out in the real world. This venting helps them be more levelheaded on the job and with their families.

I never have easy answers for clients who suffer with jealousy and envy, because I personally know how difficult these feelings are to manage. I have always admired academic brilliance, because it was such a high priority to my parents. All through school I envied others who were the top achievers in my class. When they were praised, I felt extremely envious.

Even today I struggle with envy. I am a new widow. Every married couple close to my age stirs up ugly feelings in me when I see them walking hand in hand or communicating with a simple look. I try very hard to remember the fifty-four years Lyall and I shared together, and I am truly thankful, but I miss his companionship terribly. Seeing what others continue to share makes the pain of my losses cut even deeper.

When I'm struggling with envy and jealousy, I cry out for help from God. These feelings are impossible for me to battle on my own. I also remind myself of God's power to forgive and cleanse me from any ugly feelings. Meditating on these truths helps them to sink deep down into my bones and allows the Holy Spirit to work on my emotions. I desperately need Him to touch me at this deeper level.

Gratefulness is also one of my antidotes for jealousy. At this time in my life, I am concentrating on being thankful for all the blessings God has given me: my family, my health, my work, my friends, and my complete recovery from serious surgery. In time, my emotions will find their way out of the black hole of grief, but until that day I'll strive to cultivate a thankful heart and do my best to be about His business.

3

Low Self-Esteem

Low self-esteem always produces tension. A person who doubts her own worth is in constant danger of being put under unbearable tension. Since low self-esteem probably developed during childhood, it is especially hard to combat, but there are things that can be done to bolster our self-esteem and help us lead productive, happy lives.

I had been asked to be the keynote speaker for a women's conference at a large suburban church. The pastor's wife and I met to discuss the focus of the meetings, and we were both uncertain about the direction the Lord wanted us to take. I suggested we draft a survey for the women in the church to complete, which would tell us what concerned them the most. The pastor's wife was shocked by the results of the survey. Nearly all the women listed two main problems: low self-esteem and depression.

I dreaded counseling clients with low self-esteem. They were usually angry about almost everything, and often discounted many of the ideas I offered. I can't tell you how many times I've heard, "What you say is fine for other people, but it doesn't work for me." In their minds, they are always victims.

"There were five girls in our family," Megan told me. "I don't think Mother liked me. She favored my sister who was fifteen months older because she was pretty and talented. Mom did more for all the other kids than she did for me. Now they're doing well, and my life is a mess."

Megan's sisters were paying for her counseling and wanted very much to see her helped. I sensed their genuine compassion for her. They said their mother had tried very hard to love Megan, but Megan was never satisfied. She always found something wrong with everything. Aside from Megan's perpetual complaint, the sisters perceived their family as happy and stable.

Our perception of ourselves is largely formed by what we think other people think of us. Parents or others do not have to specifically say, "You don't measure up, and you never will." In fact, those around us may go overboard to try to make us feel valued. Still, each of us has our own perception about whether we are "good" or "no good."

Eileen felt "no good." When she made an appointment with me, she was very worried because her husband wanted a legal separation. He had planned this rather carefully. Even though he was still supporting Eileen and the children, she thought he had found another woman. She desperately wanted him back, under any circumstance, partly because she didn't want to work while her children were young.

I could see why Eileen's husband might have lost interest in her. Her appearance was dowdy. She showed little awareness of the world outside her home and confined her interests to her children. I saw the danger signals flashing and was rather direct with Eileen: "You must not bank on his continued support. If indeed he is planning an escape, I doubt the money will continue to be sent. It might be good for you to think about training for a part-time job of some kind."

Eileen was fortunate to find a small local business that offered on-the-job training. A friend nearby cared for her children after school. Eileen soon discovered that she had talents that had never been tapped. The firm found her exceptionally skilled, and she loved the work. It was exciting to watch Eileen's confidence grow.

She also worked on improving her appearance. I'm a firm believer that even the most homely woman can look beautiful if she will take an interest in herself and be willing to make some necessary changes. One afternoon Eileen walked into my office without her thick glasses. She had lovely eyes, and thanks to contact lenses, I was now able to see them. She had also consulted one of the cosmetic specialists at a local mall for advice about makeup. Further advice about clothing and a growing knowledge of styles and colors made a remarkable transformation. Wherever she went, her friends said, "Eileen, you look great! I've never seen you look better."

The positive feedback made Eileen feel better about herself, despite her husband's desertion. Her confidence grew, and she began to realize that even if her husband did go through with the divorce, she could make it and life would be all right.

After a few months, Eileen's husband started paying frequent visits to the house and began to show interest in Eileen. One Wednesday night she was gone during his regular visit. The following day he called to inquire where she had been. I suggested this might happen and that she should seem a bit mysterious. Prepared, she said, "Oh, I was just out. I have a lot of things going on right now."

Soon he suggested they try courting again and plan a date each week. Eventually he asked her if he could come home. Because Eileen's self-esteem had improved over the months, she was able to say to him, "I'm not sure that your coming home is best for me and the children right now. I will not be treated like a doormat any longer. I have needs that must be respected if we are to have a future together." With new ground rules for the relationship, he eventually moved home, and their marriage is stronger than ever.

I realize that every story doesn't have such a happy ending. However, Eileen improved her self-esteem in a short period of time, and this affected her and her marriage for good. I'm certain it influenced her job satisfaction and success, too.

If we aren't appealing to ourselves, we are certainly not going to find others attracted to us. We must find things that spark our interest, especially those of us who are prone to constantly give to others at our own expense. Now don't get me wrong; I believe and practice servanthood, but if we are constantly giving and never nourishing ourselves, our self-esteem will suffer. We must develop interests we can call our own. I learned more about this from Jenny, as she sat in her wheelchair telling me about one of the loves of her life.

For many years she had been a shut-in. It wasn't only the crippling disease that confined her to her home; it was partly her poor self-esteem. She hated being pitied by onlookers.

One day a friend gave her a charming little bell. Her family members noticed the joy this brought her and made a point of giving her other bells on special occasions. Jenny's new interest led her to study bells from all over the world. She gathered unique stories about them and was eventually asked to speak at women's retreats about her rare collection. She became an authority on bells and was offered many invitations to speak to various groups. There was no more confinement and self-absorption, no more low self-esteem for Jenny.

One young woman I know married a man whose position in the political arena required them to entertain national and international tradesmen. One evening her husband said, "I would like you to study the expansion of Japanese exports and imports, especially in the car industry. I don't have the time, and it will keep the conversation going when we take officials to dinner."

This intelligent woman disciplined herself and studied the topic. In time she was well-versed in Japanese trade expansion. At a luncheon with some business guests, one of them asked her husband a specific question about the effect of Japanese trade on the banking systems in the United States. He replied, "Oh, that is of great interest to my wife. She's the specialist in this area. Let's ask her."

She later told me that all the guests wanted to discuss the topic and she knew more about the issue than anyone in the room. The conversation continued for over an hour.

"I have never felt better about myself!" she exclaimed to me.

This woman didn't suffer feelings of inferiority prior to her husband's request, but her ability to converse about Japanese trade gave her a feeling of confidence she had not known before.

I remember many years ago, when I spoke for the first time at a very large church. I had been asked to address the Sunday evening service. I accepted the church's invitation, figuring Sunday evening services weren't especially well attended. I didn't realize that the senior pastor had publicized the service as an outreach opportunity. My topic for the evening was, "How can a man understand a woman?" He had encouraged the congregation to invite friends, neighbors, and couples who were having marital difficulties.

When I arrived at the church, I discovered they wanted me to march onto the platform and sit with the pastors at the beginning of the service. I wasn't used to this kind of arrangement but went along with it, not wanting to rock the boat. I walked onto the platform in that tremendous auditorium and could see there was standing room only. I literally panicked. I got up and sat with the congregation. Shaking with fear, I wanted more than anything to escape. Sitting beside the head of women's ministries, I kept trying to think of ways I could bow out of the occasion graciously. Just before the pastor turned the service over to me, the dear lady next to me said, "Remember, Jean, you know more about your subject than anyone else in the entire church, including all those pastors up there. You are the specialist!"

That's all it took to calm me down so I could face the task ahead. Plodding up the platform stairs, I felt overwhelmed with the assignment, but her words bolstered my self-esteem and gave me courage to do the job God wanted me to do. Since that time I've had the privilege of speaking to thousands of people across the nation. Sometimes the jitters still get the best of me, especially when the crowds are so big that I can't see the faces in the audience. But those encouraging words from years ago continue to help me when I'm feeling insecure: "Remember, Jean, you're the specialist."

Become a specialist in one small area that interests you. Work at it. Learn all you can about it. It will make a difference in how you feel about yourself and how others perceive you.

The Pain of Perfectionism

As difficult as it is to believe, perfectionists suffer from low self-esteem. In order to like themselves, they must be perfect. Unfortunately, they can't be perfect, and this failing reinforces their low self-esteem. It's a vicious circle.

She whizzed by me, walking as fast as her long legs would allow. "Good morning, Mrs. Lee," I called. "I haven't seen you for a few days."

Doing an about-face, she darted toward me with a pressured stride. "I've been terribly busy from morning to night," she said. "All Jack's golf buddies and their wives are in town, and it's my turn to entertain. Thank God I don't have to do this very often!"

As she stopped to catch her breath, I said, "Your home and garden always look beautiful. I can't imagine there would be much preparation for your company."

Shocked, she retorted, "Oh my! There is so much work to be done. I've just finished giving the gardener precise directions on how to lay the fresh pea gravel in the paths. I'm sure I'll have to rake the gravel just before our guests arrive."

"But your garden always looks beautiful, with its lovely pink petunia borders."

"It's not perfect, by any means! You can see that all the petunias aren't the exact same shade of pink. I wanted everything to match perfectly, but the greenhouse erred on my order this year. I would have refused to purchase these flowers, but they were the only pink petunias left in town, and I had to have something to put along the path for this weekend."

"Oh, Mrs. Lee, your house looks beautiful, and I admire the way your whole family works with you to keep it so lovely."

"Well, thank you, but I can't stand here talking. The party is tomorrow, and I'm a nervous wreck. I hate the way these parties interfere with my routine." Shaking her head, she headed toward her house. "I've got to go. There's laundry and ironing to do."

"Couldn't you hide the laundry until after the party?" I called. In total amazement, she peered at me, her eyes as big as quarters. "I could never do that! I can't stand having soiled articles in my house. What if someone found them?"

I was just a young mother when I lived next door to Mrs. Lee, and I remember leaving that conversation feeling like a downright failure. At the time I had never heard the word *perfectionist*. I just thought she was a wonderful manager and housekeeper, and I wished my house looked as lovely as hers.

Mrs. Lee was meticulous about tiny details, always straining for excellence, but even her highest standards weren't good enough. She always felt she had to be better. Not only was she worn out, but she was wearing out her husband and children, too. Whenever her sense of order was disturbed, they caught the flack.

It goes without saying that perfectionists are often angry people. They usually carry low-grade irritation inside, because nothing measures up to their expectations. They expect too much out of themselves, out of others, and even out of God. It's interesting to me that out of the ten personality types, perfectionists have the highest rate of depression.[1]

Sloppy people are sometimes happier. They don't get so frustrated when things aren't in complete order. Now I don't advocate living in a pigpen, but perhaps we would enjoy life more if we weren't so uptight about having everything spotless.

Deborah was a perfectionistic housewife who worked part time and was involved in the women's ministry at her church.

"I love all the things I do," Deborah sighed, "but I'm not juggling the load well. Something is wrong with me. Plenty of my friends do more than me, and yet they're calm and relaxed. I'm anything but calm. It's like I have a knot in my throat all the time."

After we explored her various responsibilities, I suggested that Deborah separate out the things that were of vital importance each day. She was to choose three areas that needed an A performance. If she listed ten priorities for the day, only the top three were to get an A performance. The other seven had to be given a B or C. I could tell she had trouble separating the urgent from the trivial.

"Make your bedroom look tidy in a few minutes, instead of fiddling around for thirty minutes doing everything perfectly," I suggested. "Give yourself permission to do it quickly. Stop dead in your tracks when your ten minutes are up, and go on to the next thing on the list. If your bedroom gets a C for the day, don't worry about it. It's okay. Push your shoes and slippers into the closet and throw up the bedcovers in two full sweeps. Forget about tucking in everything. A C on your bedroom doesn't matter when you have other important deadlines to meet. Leave the dishes in the dishwasher unwashed, and don't vacuum before going to work. We are doing this to get you away from living to perfectionistic extremes."

I don't think I gained her confidence very quickly, because she scoffed, "That's awful. I will never stoop to such sloppy housekeeping!"

I tried to reason with her. "You have just told me that you are perpetually exhausted. You have also told me that you have important deadlines to meet at certain times of the month and on those days you have to be out of the house very early. You cannot assign A grades to every single task each day. If you do, you're going to be a neurotic mess. You must learn to separate out the most important tasks."

She reluctantly agreed to try the plan I offered and wrote out her schedule for the following day. At first she assigned too many Bs after her top three A tasks. Gradually she worked on accepting more Cs in the plan. When she came in the next week, I asked for every detail.

"As soon as I started sensing the knot in my throat, I talked to myself. Last night we entertained eight dinner guests, and I told myself I must not demand perfection in every part of the house. I let the basement stay as it was and told the children they had to keep the doors to their rooms closed. The kids' toys were strewn all over the family room floor, so I closed it off, too. I vacuumed the house the day before and gave myself permission to leave the Hoover in the closet until after the party. I decided the dining room and kitchen would get the A grade for the evening, along with the meal I prepared."

"Excellent!" I said. "But how did you feel about all the neglect?"

I smiled inside when I heard Deborah's response.

"Jean, it was kind of weird. I really enjoyed the evening with our friends. I've never found entertaining pleasurable, because all the preparation wore me out. But last night was different. I actually had fun, and it was great to hear everyone rave about the stuffed chicken breasts."

Then a strange thing happened that caught me totally off guard. Without warning, she shouted at the top of her voice, "Mother, I don't *have* to be *perfect anymore*! I can't please you, anyway! I refuse to feel guilty for not being what you have always pushed me to be!"

Deborah's mother had been dead for several years.

Living Below Our Potential

After many years in a counseling office, I am convinced that living below one's potential is both a cause and effect of tension. When we have a potential of 160 points and are living at a reality of 100 points, we know we are not living up to our potential, and our self-esteem suffers another blow, leading to constant tension and depression.

I've heard hundreds of women despair about chronic pressure. They feel trapped by circumstances completely beyond their control. They mourn the passing years while dreaming of what they could be doing with their talents and abilities. They have no time, no energy, and no drive to be involved in something that could pull them out of their depression. Even survival seems hard.

Existential psychologist A. H. Maslow made a significant statement: "All human beings must seek their God-given mission in their lifetime, and in the search therein lies their identity." He didn't say this based on a Christian belief system. He proposed it simply as a basic principle of good mental health, but his idea parallels what Scripture teaches: God has a plan for each of us.

I want to tell you about God's plan for my precious sister. Discovering her God-given mission literally transformed her life. She was a frail child, born prematurely and almost fatally poisoned by a formula she was fed. This left her in a very delicate state. As a young child, she was attacked by polio and suffered a very long recovery period. During her illness she wasn't allowed to attend school, and this was a blow to her self-esteem. She also lived in a household that was intellectually threatening to her.

After we were grown and away from home, my sister confided to me that she had felt like a failure while growing up. She felt Mother and Father preferred me over her because I was assertive and intellectual, whereas she was gentle and didn't aspire to the goals valued by our parents. I was shocked to learn that she had suffered terribly with depression when she was sixteen.

My sister married a dear, gentle, Christian man who had a similar background. He never functioned well in the competitive world and became very dependent on her. Much of this was due to the severe health problems he had endured all his life.

After marriage, my sister's life was confined to her small home. Most of the time she felt she shouldn't leave her invalid husband unattended. She wanted to be involved in church activities, but regular attendance wasn't always possible.

The Lord heard the cry of her heart. One night as they were preparing for bed, the senior pastor of her church called. He told my sister that he and his wife had suddenly been called to a tragic emergency, and they needed someone to care for their three children. An elder had suggested my sister because of her talent with small children.

That was just the beginning. The Lord began to show her that she had a unique ministry to pastoral families because she was always home. For years she made herself available in emergencies to the five ministers of that church who were raising youngsters.

My sister found meaning and fulfillment in her ministry. As far as I know, she gave her time joyfully and never received payment for her services, but the rewards went far beyond any dollar figure.

I cannot imagine being on call like my sister. Her mission in life would drive me bonkers. And she cannot imagine doing what I do. She'd likely have cardiac arrest if someone asked her to stand in front of large crowds to teach. God knows this. That's why He designs a mission to perfectly fit our lifestyle, our personality, and our experience. He will only ask us to do what He equips us to do—nothing more, nothing less.

My good friend Susan Bailey found this to be true in her life, too. Susan grew up on a farm in South Australia and was forced to drop out of school when she was fourteen, due to tuberculosis. Her health was frail for several years, but eventually she was able to do light domestic work. She and I became Christians about the same time and attended the same fellowship group. She met Bill in the group, and later they married.

Susan and Bill were extremely active in their suburban church and thrived on their interactions with others, but after about a year, Susan's health began to fail. Her doctor advised them to move away from the heat on the plains to the hill country, a few miles from where they lived.

In the hill country there was only one church, and it was spiritually dead. One roving minister looked after five tiny churches on a circuit, holding Sunday service in their church every now and then. Susan was particularly discouraged about the spiritual deadness in the church. She began to pray faithfully each day for change. After several weeks passed, Susan and Bill met two other young couples who agreed to come to their house to pray on Wednesday nights. Together they implored God to send them a minister who was spiritually on fire and would commit himself to the church.

Well, a new minister did come to the church, but he wasn't exactly what they requested. He was a sick, beaten-down missionary sent home to rest. After this weary missionary was at the church a few weeks, Susan invited him to their prayer meeting, hoping their prayers would encourage him. He didn't go at the time, but several months later, he suddenly felt compelled to attend the prayer meeting. He knew the time and place, so without informing anyone, he went.

There was a long footpath up to Susan and Bill's front door. Hearing the group in the middle of their prayers, the pastor walked very quietly up to the house. It was a hot, still summer night, and the doors and windows were open to catch the passing breezes. His ears perked up when his name was mentioned: "Oh, God, please restore Reverend Brown's body to good health and stir up his soul so he will know how to preach the gospel again. Oh, Lord, he is so dead, and so discouraged, and we're getting depressed, too. We keep beseeching You to change him, but nothing is happening. Please help us, God."

The Reverend Kenneth Brown stood behind the door, not knowing what to do. Eventually he went inside and joined the group. They never knew until months later that he heard their prayers, but after that, he faithfully attended the prayer meeting.

One Wednesday night the pastor said, "I have an idea for the church to consider. Our regular Sunday morning meeting is not growing. People come in and sleep through the service. It's time for something new. There are five churches in this circuit, with many teenagers who need to know about the love of God. I want to have a camp meeting just for teenagers. I've been given permission by the authorities to use the agriculture fairgrounds. We can bed everyone down in the straw, but I'll need a lot of help to run the camp. Would you team up with me? How about it?"

The results were phenomenal! Reverend Brown preached about God's love to the teens in a new and fearless way. His soul caught fire for God, and the camp meetings marked the beginning of an awakening in all five of his churches.

What happened to Bill and Susan? Their dreams materialized when they became missionaries in the interior of Australia.

Despite frail health, and no education or outstanding talent, Susan was mightily used by God in a dynamic ministry.

Sometimes I think we cop out and say God can't use us because we aren't especially talented or educated. God isn't concerned about our capabilities—all He wants is our availability. He asks us to offer what we have. When we do the possible, He does the impossible.

Most of us have times when we don't like ourselves. Perhaps we were conditioned during childhood to believe we were less important than others. Maybe we've tried to cover our inadequacies by striving for perfection, which makes us weary but not confident. We can't change the events of our childhood or the people around us, but we can always make the choice to improve ourselves. We can develop interests. We can take time to listen to God. I love what Robert Browning said: "My business is not to remake myself, but to make the absolute best of what God has made."[2] Discovering His mission for our lives boosts our self-esteem more than anything else this world has to offer.

4
Grief

Anyone suffering from grief is under tension. There's no way around that. The trick is to deal with our grief in a healthy manner, knowing it will pass with time, and not allow it to warp our lives.

Many years ago, a teenager named Kelly was assigned to me at the counseling agency. Kelly's foster mother was having severe difficulties with her. Kelly's grades were failing at school, and nothing seemed to motivate her. We knew she was intelligent from a battery of tests, but her behavior didn't match her aptitude. I was given the job of finding the reason for her poor performance and helping her improve scholastically. From her file, I learned that her mother had been killed in a car accident when Kelly was six.

During Kelly's first session with me, I wanted to hear about her past. I was utterly startled when she said, "Well, for starters, I killed my mother when I was six years old."

"How can this be?" I replied. "Your mother was killed in a car accident, when you weren't there."

"No, you don't understand!" she protested. "She wasn't really killed by the car. The day before the accident, I was furious with her and said, 'I hope you die tomorrow, because I hate you!' My wish killed her. Don't try to persuade me otherwise. I know in my heart that I killed her."

Kelly sincerely believed she alone caused her mother's death and she deserved nothing good for the rest of her life. She had turned all her anger over her mother's death onto herself. I worked hard to help Kelly let go of the anger-induced tension that was ruining her life.

Sometimes we're angry at ourselves when someone we love dies, and sometimes our tension comes out as anger at the person who died. A close friend of mine lost her husband very suddenly. He was perfectly well one minute and dead the next.

Carol is one of the most saintly women I have ever known. After her husband's death, she appeared to cope with great peace. There was no hysteria, no panic, and no dysfunctional reactions.

Some months later, when we were sharing a pot of tea, she leaned toward me and said, "You know, I suppose I'm awful for thinking this, but I have been so angry with Art. How could he go and die on me and leave me with all these problems to face alone?"

She was so apologetic about her feelings and guilty for even having them. I jumped at the opportunity to explain that her anger was a normal part of grief and that I was relieved she could recognize and acknowledge her feelings so clearly.

Sandra Aldrich, another friend of mine from the Focus on the Family staff, lost her husband in the prime of life. In a recent interview, she spoke of the bewildering anger she experienced after Don's death:

I didn't know anger could take so many forms. I felt God's presence during Don's illness and immediately after his death, so I panicked when I thought God had left me alone in later months. Feeling spiritually abandoned, I demanded, "Why aren't You talking to me?"

Suddenly I thought of times when I had held an injured Jay or Holly on my lap. I hadn't talked, but had merely held them against my heart, surrounding hurt with love. I realized what the Lord was doing for me.

I was also angry about relatives who ignored opportunities to encourage him, and me, through visits, calls, and offers of practical help. It would have been nice if someone had offered to take our children to the park. The only way I could get rid of that anger was by facing it and sobbing it out in prayer. It also helped to remember times when I had undoubtedly been ignorant of their pain as well.

Especially hurtful were the remarks they made at the funeral home when they told me how much they had loved Don and how his courage had helped them. I wondered why they had never bothered telling him those things *before* he died. Forgiving them, even when they hadn't asked me to, was the only thing that helped.

I remember flaring up in anger when I witnessed indifference or rudeness between couples. As husbands and wives argued over petty things, I wanted to yell, "Don't you know what you have?" But I said nothing, knowing I wouldn't have listened years ago either.

Jean, I really didn't want to be angry because it zapped my energy that could be better used someplace else. But sometimes I couldn't help it. It's nice to know emotions aren't right or wrong; they just are. So I just try to handle them the best I can whenever they come.[1]

During personal grief, I've found it helpful to read the accounts of others who have known pain. How did they manage? What enabled them to cope with the heartache that

words can't describe? I've asked several individuals who have journeyed through the valley of death to contribute to this chapter. They will share with you some of their challenges and triumphs. As you enter their world, look for nuggets to set aside for a day when you may need them.

Empty Arms
(Pam Vredevelt)

"I'm not picking up a heartbeat, Pam. There doesn't appear to be any fetal movement. I think the baby is dead."

In disbelief my emotions began to run wild and unchecked. Engulfed in a jumble of scrambled thoughts, I wanted desperately to hear the doctor say, "Wait a minute—I'm wrong. I've made a mistake. Now I see the heartbeat." Those words never came.

During the next half hour in that little examining room, my life was a blur. Everything was out of focus. I hated my humanness. "Why can't I change this and make things different?" I thought. Somehow I wanted to say a few words and magically raise our baby from the dead.

Nothing made sense. Angry questions darted back and forth in my mind. "Why is this happening to me? To John? It's not fair! Thousands have abortions, but we want this child . . . why are we the ones to get ripped off? I hate this!"

For years we had ministered to others in the counseling office and at church who were suffering grief. Now it was our turn to experience it. Emotions raced in and out without any logical progression. We couldn't keep up with them. At those times we talked to ourselves out loud. We reminded our intellects that these grief feelings were normal. We weren't unspiritual to feel them. We weren't going off the deep end. We were merely walking the road of healing.

The journey through our grief was not easy, but we did gain some insights along the way. We learned to relax with the penetrating truth that life has surprises that are above and beyond our control. Growth came as we adjusted to our unexpected jolt and invested time in understanding ourselves, each other, and God.

We were forced to look death squarely in the face. This deepened our appreciation for the sanctity of life. We learned to embrace pain, anger, guilt, and sadness. This enriched our understanding of our humanity and deepened our intimacy with God. In the midst of our heartache we learned it was better to pursue wisdom than to look for pat answers. Our healing was a process, not an instantaneous event. And in that process we discovered some tools that helped us toward personal growth. I have included more about surviving the loss of a baby in my book, *Empty Arms: Emotional Support for Those Who Have Suffered Miscarriage or Stillbirth.*

One of the most helpful things we learned came from Sharon, the nurse who talked with me during the moments following the doctor's announcement that our baby was dead. She said, "We live in a fallen world and sometimes the pain and suffering of this fallen world touches our lives. It isn't fair, I know, but nothing will be totally fair and perfect until we get to heaven."

Our loss has taught me that because this world is fallen, I must learn to expect the innocent to sometimes be victims of heartache. Losses aren't a sign of sin in my life or a message from God to "shape up my act." Losses are simply a form of suffering common to the human experience of living in this world. Not everything in life is fair or predictable. Many wrongs are not made right. Yet there will be a day when a final judgment will be made, and at that time everything will be set straight. Until that time I must accept the fact that I will go through times when my human experience is painful. There will be times when I have questions and no answers. There will be times when heartache will be hard to bear. This is part of living in a fallen world.

While I accept this fact, I can at the same time have hope for bright tomorrows. I know without a doubt that "in all things God works for the good of those who love him" (Rom. 8:28). Some people may read this verse and interpret it this way: God works pain and joy, good and evil into my life for my good. Thus miscarriage, stillbirth, or any other loss is inflicted upon me by God in order to accomplish good in my life. I prefer to look at it another way. God did not afflict us with the death of our baby to work a certain "good" or growth into our lives. Rather, our lives were touched by the pain of human experience, and in the process of groping for answers and understanding, growth was produced. God's involvement with us in that growth process gave us hope, strength, tenacity, and comfort. As we came to grips with our anger and depression and guilt, God stepped into our human weakness and lifted us out of the depths of despair. That is how God worked good into our lives during our loss.

Jesus said, "I have told you these things, so that in me you may have peace. In this world you will have trouble. But take heart! I have overcome the world" (John 16:33). God knew we would experience the sting of pain and suffering. With that understanding, He offers the encouraging words that He has "overcome the world." So in the midst of my humanness, He can reach into my life and help me stand on my feet again. He brings peace to my turmoil. He brings order to my chaos. He brings hope to my despair. Truly God is a good God.[2]

I Wish Others Knew
(Sandra Aldrich)

The day our doctor told us Ken's diagnosis, I had no idea how my love for God would be tested. I remember kneeling with Ken the following evening at a prayer meeting, with pastors hovering over us. Weeping, I prayed, "It's okay, Lord. I trust Your sovereignty." I later told my sister about my prayer and asked her to remind me of it, if I said something to the contrary. But, she never did.

Nothing prepared me for his bout with leukemia and his death. I didn't know I would feel like I had undergone an emotional amputation. It's like part of me has been cut away forever. I didn't know how endlessly the future would stretch before me, at least not until the day I met an eighty-five-year-old widow whose mate had died thirty years earlier when she was my age. That was when hopelessness numbed me.

When Ken first died, I was outraged. How dare God take him? I felt God owed me an apology. I am still miffed about it, but the pity parties are fewer and further between. I didn't feel angry with Ken for the first six months after the funeral. Then one day when I was mowing the lawn, I was so weary with the task that I stopped the mower, looked up to heaven, and screamed at Ken for abandoning me. I still resent being left with all the jobs he used to do for me. Putting up the Christmas tree usually calls for a good speech!

To my dismay, there have been many surprises. I haven't been a pillar of strength. It has been five years since the funeral, and I still wonder if there will ever be a day when I'll awake in the morning and my first thoughts won't be of Ken. I still have sudden urges to call him about something nice that has happened, like a good job review, the announcement of a new grandbaby, or my purchase of a new dress. I desperately miss our daily prayer times together and the intimacy we shared as husband and wife. My mind says, "I surrendered Ken to God many years ago." Yet my heart remains entwined in the cords of love that bonded us together during his time on earth.

I feel a social void because most of my free time is spent strictly with women. I enjoy being with men, too, but there are few mixed activities for those who aren't couples. Even at family events I feel somewhat like a fifth wheel.

Fear rears its ugly head, too. Fear of failure. Fear I won't be able to manage the small inheritance Ken left me. Fear of not being taken care of should I become ill. I think it was Benson who said, "The worst sorrows in life are not in its losses and misfortunes, but in its fears." I agree.

During the last five years I have become painfully aware that I am not the fine example of victorious widowhood I had imagined I would be the day Ken died. I am not helpful to others in my situation. In my tear- and coffee-stained Bible that we carried in our car for years, I highlighted Psalm 69:6, "May those who hope in you not be disgraced because of me, O Lord, the Lord Almighty; may those who seek you not be put to shame because of me." In the margin next to it I penned, "God, please don't let me be an embarrassment to You or to my family. Don't let people stumble because of my reactions to what You have permitted in my life."

I do believe I will not make further progress in my emotional healing nor in my relationship with God until I accept the fact that I am forgiven. I've asked God to forgive me for wanting an apology from Him for Ken's death. In my weariness I've said, "God, I am willing to be willing to smile again. I want to know joy on a daily basis and to feel like I am useful again. Do Your work in me."

I wish people knew that I like hearing Ken's name mentioned. So many try to pretend he didn't exist, for fear I'll dissolve into tears if they talk about him. I wish people knew that just because I look okay doesn't mean I am okay. I still hurt. Several years have passed since he died, but that doesn't mean time has healed all wounds.

I wish people knew that I love hearing how they miss Ken. I wish they knew the joy I feel when he is quoted at church, or when I'm told that his taped sermons continue to be an encouragement. Knowing his influence has not died seems to make the letting go a little easier.[3]

54

I Needed Forgiveness
(Neta Jackson)

Setting out from Seattle it was still dark, and I was a bit apprehensive about the long drive ahead of me. I had never driven across the country before. But we were moving Mom and Dad to Chicago to be closer to the rest of the family. They needed me to drive their car for them.

By the end of the first day my confidence was up and I was actually enjoying being the principal driver. My eighty-two-year-old father seemed to enjoy riding shotgun, while Mom sat in the backseat pointing out the beauty of the country around us.

The second day we traveled the empty Montana interstate. Later in the afternoon I noticed my dad was leaning awkwardly sideways as he napped. I reached behind the front seat for a pillow to prop him up. Suddenly I realized the car was drifting off the road. I jerked the steering wheel, but the car spun out of control, flew off the road at sixty miles per hour, rolled once, and landed backward in the ditch below.

"What have I done? What have I done?" I cried. As the dust settled I could see the car was demolished.

"What happened?" my mother said in a frail voice from the backseat. She assured me she was all right, then leaned up to check on Daddy. He was leaning toward me in his seat belt with his eyes open, trying to speak. But no words came out. Then he closed his eyes.

Panicking, I climbed out my broken window and ran up to the road to flag down help. A car and a truck stopped. They helped my mother out of our car and wrapped her in a blanket. But Dad just lay on the front seat, his eyes closed.

Pacing back and forth, all I could say was, "I've killed my dad . . . I've killed my dad." I reached through the driver's window, placed my hand on his head, and frantically prayed, "Oh, God, don't let him die . . . please don't let my dad die." Somehow I sensed my prayer was in vain.

An ambulance transported Dad to the hospital. When the police car delivered us to the emergency room, we heard the news that Dad had died of a heart attack. I had let my entire family down. And God had let me down.

People were kind, saying, "It's not your fault. He didn't die of injuries. He might have died of a heart attack, even without an accident . . . don't blame yourself. You were only trying to help him." No one blamed me, but I blamed myself.

While we waited at the hospital for relatives to arrive, a local pastor came to our side and stayed for hours. This stranger sat with his arm around me. My shoulder was bruised and his hug hurt, but I didn't tell him. I needed to be held. "I feel like I've killed my dad!" I said in broken words between sobs.

He didn't reassure me. He didn't blame me. He said, "It sounds like you need to be forgiven."

Yes. That was what I needed. To whatever degree I was responsible for the accident, I did not need assurance that I was blameless, but forgiveness. While holding me, he led me in prayer asking God's forgiveness.

But the question remained. Why had God let me down? During the months that followed I asked God to help me understand, and some new thoughts came to mind.

Perhaps He had answered my prayer. Mom and I were not hurt in the crash. All three of us had been wearing seat belts and only received minor cuts and bruises. Those who later saw the car wondered how anyone walked away alive. Even though we were far from home, the accident happened only one hundred miles from my father's boyhood home. He was buried in the same country cemetery next to his father, mother, sister, and brother. This had been his wish for years.

And Dad suffered no pain. He died vigorous and healthy. Just that morning in our motel room I woke up to him doing pushups. I had always hoped he wouldn't suffer a long illness before his death.

Dad had lived long enough to help Mom sell the house, arrange for a retirement community, and pack for the move. Everything had been accomplished, and he looked forward to some deserved rest.

For months flashbacks of the car hurtling off the road haunted me. I couldn't think of Dad without replaying the accident. On the year anniversary of Dad's death, as the hour of the accident approached, feelings of agitation escalated within me. Leaving the house in a flurry, I bundled my jacket against the crisp October wind and went to a nearby park. Sitting on a bench I remembered and cried, remembered and cried. I'm not sure why, but I seemed to turn a corner that day. From that point on I was able to think about Dad without the horrifying flashbacks.

Sometimes I still wonder why and how it happened. Dad had noticed a shimmy in the wheels earlier that day. Had a tire blown? I don't know. And I will never know the answers to these questions. But I do know that I've been forgiven for my inability to safely drive my parents to Chicago. And Dad? Well, he's getting the much-deserved rest he wanted, and experiencing heavenly wonders I can only anticipate.[4]

Final Thoughts about Grief

I always knew I could face anything in life, as long as my husband was with me. Nothing was more important to me than Lyall.

It was easy for me to give up everything else to be home for him. I was thankful we could manage caring for him at home. His illness did take its toll on me physically, but I didn't mind.

The day of Pa's memorial service, I awoke in the early hours of the morning and opened my Bible and daily devotional to read. I was amazed at the verse in the heading of a devotional: "The hand of the Lord hath wrought this" (Job 12:9).

Sometimes we do experience a terrible blow, and perhaps it is so sudden that we feel it is undeserved, unfair, and unjust. All we can feel is that this blow is a mistake God is making in our lives, but if only we knew that this was to be the beginning of a new refining of our souls.

God can make something of us as we endure the discipline and take the shaping as He makes us afresh. It is much like a gem cutter who must take the roughest sort of rock and, with calculated hammer blows and the work of fine chisels, produces a beautiful gem that otherwise would have been buried forever.

I was saying to God, "What's the use of my living, now that You have taken the most important person in my life away from me? How can I cope? How can I go on? I can't! And Lord, did You ever think of the children and the grandchildren when you took Lyall away? He was their security, too."

The anger came in waves. The tears flowed. I had never wept as I have during this year. I suppose Poppa's death has tapped into all the other anger and grief I've suffered during the rest of my life. My daughter asked me if I had ever grieved when my brother died in his youth or when my parents died, or when my first grandson died. I had to answer no.

Poppa's death unleashed a reservoir of grief that had collected throughout my entire lifetime. I read an article by a biochemist recently that seemed to confirm this. Dr. William Frey, who has studied the hormonal component of tears, says that in relation to grief, "These tears have often been hidden for years. They are not usually tears for the present, but for what has been in the past."[5]

What is the solution to this kind of deep suffering? I don't have a magical cure, but I can pass on some of the things that have helped me the most. First, recognize that anger is a big part of grief. It's perfectly natural, and must not be denied. It is healthy to feel the anger. Don't try to be superspiritual, thinking you must live up to some kind of image you have created in your mind. You will pay a high price for denial and rigid control of your emotions.

Second, accept your anger without feeling guilty. Understand that experts in grief therapy are more concerned about those who don't feel anger when they are grieving than those who do.

Third, let the tears flow. As Dr. Frey says, "Don't stifle your tears. Allow them to wash away the stress."

Finally, express your anger in constructive ways. Perhaps you can begin by talking to God. He already knows what you are feeling, and He will not be offended. He loves you unconditionally and wants to help carry the burden of your grief. God is no security against storms, but He is perfect security in storms. He never promised us an easy passage, only a safe landing. In the midst of my grief, I'm sensing the security and safety God can give. Remember, God isn't partial; He'll help you as He has helped me. You need only ask.

5

Recapitulation

Most of us occasionally rehash various incidents in our lives, especially those that were painful. There are, however, certain times when being obsessed with the past is more common, particularly when we endure a trauma, a prolonged period of stress, or a hormonal shift. This tendency to relive the past is called recapitulation, and it only brings us more tension.

"It's been three years since that creep walked out on me, and I'm as angry today as I was the day it happened!" Dorothy cried. "Every time I think about that younger woman, I want to kill her. What did I do to deserve this? How did I lose him to that predator? Didn't I love him enough? Did I love him too much? How could I have been so foolish and blind? So stupid! My friends warned me, but I thought they were crazy. Why, oh why, didn't I listen to them? If only I had. . . ."

Dorothy was a middle-aged woman who wanted help dealing with her anger. Ever since her divorce, she'd felt as if she were wired differently. The slightest provocation sent her into a rage. As she shared her deepest feelings with me, I could tell she was stuck recapitulating, obsessing about the past. Over and over she relived her husband leaving her for his young secretary, and with each review, surges of angry hatred burst to the surface.

Dorothy had endured a trauma and a prolonged period of stress. The divorce was a long, drawn-out process with an ugly custody battle. Her husband not only wanted to trade her in for a sleek young woman, he wanted to take the kids with him!

There were other pressures on Dorothy. Her aging parents lived in the same town and depended heavily on her. The same year her husband left, her oldest daughter left for college and her youngest son turned thirteen. Now she had to contend with the grief caused by her husband and firstborn leaving, while trying to parent two teenagers.

Dorothy was also experiencing many symptoms characteristic of thirty-eight- to forty-three-year-old women. This is the time of life when a woman's body goes through hormonal shifts as the reproductive system begins gearing down. For some women, these symptoms pass quickly. For others, they continue for a couple years. Dorothy's symptoms lingered, and undoubtedly the shock of her husband's affair and the divorce proceedings made things worse. Dorothy isn't alone.

Many happily married and single women between thirty-eight and forty-three speak of a strong tendency to recapitulate. I believe this is hormone related. They look at the past and hate themselves for what they did or didn't do. I've heard it time and again: "If I only knew then what I know now." "I wish I could have a second chance." "Why wasn't I more assertive?" "Why didn't I keep quiet?"

Further, recapitulation doesn't stop with what we didn't do. It goes on to include regrets over what we did do, along with every injustice others ever inflicted upon us.

I've seen women during this phase of life get so stuck obsessing about the past that they were unable to function. It reminds me of dogs that thoroughly chew bones, bury them, then later dig them up to gnaw some more.

I think men have an advantage over women when it comes to putting regrets behind them. I remember a man who was absolutely crushed because his wife and children had left him. He was suicidal, and serious about shooting himself. He actually brought the gun with him to his first appointment and fiddled with it on his lap while we talked. Yes, I was tense. I took the necessary precautions to ensure our safety, but the case worried me the rest of the week. I diligently prayed for that man each day, and hoped he would return for his next appointment.

A week later I dreaded seeing him again, but was relieved to find him alive and unarmed. He came into my office, sat down very jauntily, and said, "Guess what? I've decided to take a job in Alaska. And I can't wait to get on with it."

I said, "Oh. I can't quite catch up with you. Last week you were dying of a broken heart and were intent on shooting yourself."

He looked at me, quite surprised, and said, "That was last week."

I was left gasping. This man left my office the same way he came in, happy and ready to go, eager to begin his new life. I marveled at the way his emotions quickly lined up behind his decision. For some reason men seem to be able to say, "This is my decision, and that's that," and then proceed unhampered by shilly-shallying emotions.

I envy this ability, and I know a lot of women who would pay big money to acquire this skill, but for most women, this won't happen. I don't care how big or little the decision is, we usually stew over it before and after the decision is made. We go back and forth, wondering if we've made the right decision, feeling insecure and unsettled. There is often a gap between our decisions and our emotions. Some may chide me for this conclusion, but I think this is just a natural part of being a woman. I see this as more pronounced during the malaise period of midlife, when a woman's body is gearing down toward the termination of her reproductive cycle.

Recapitulation seems to be more extreme during menopause and after any surgery that affects the reproductive system. I have heard women report severe emotional problems six months to two years after a hysterectomy. Many of their doctors had reassured them, saying, "You'll feel wonderful—like a new woman—after the surgery." Yet not all women do. Some report severe bouts of depression and weird mood swings. Many get stuck in a recapitulation phase, dredging up things from their past. Others suffer panic attacks and feel they are going crazy.

Unexpected trauma, prolonged periods of stress, midlife malaise, and menopause can trigger recapitulation. Sometimes just plain aging can do so, too. The natural process of slowing down and having more time to think can lead us to review the past. Sometimes those glances over our shoulder are pleasurable, but for those who have lived difficult lives, recapitulation will bring pain, anger, and tension.

There have been times in my own life when I've been bogged down in a quagmire of the "if onlys." My own recapitulations brought on lingering depressions that left me feeling mentally and spiritually paralyzed. I remember the long recovery after a hysterectomy, when I was obsessed about my relationship with my mother. For years I bottled up things that I wanted to say to her. I couldn't express how much I loved her. I wished that I had understood her better. She needed me and the rest of the children to appreciate and encourage her.

There were many "if onlys." If only I had understood her needs. If only I hadn't been so emotionally controlled. If only I had expressed more affection. How different things could have been.

One of our children eloped, dropping out of college and abandoning a scholarship. Many times I have recapitulated over that. "Why did we allow her to work away from home that summer? What was lacking in our relationship? Why did she feel we were too poor to help her through college? Was I too critical at the time? Did we expect too much of her? Was I treating her the way my mother treated me?" The questions were repeated time and again in my mind.

Why did I allow my husband to drag us away from Australia? For many years I wanted Lyall's decisions to be right. When I was uneasy about something he wanted to do, I chided myself for not being a supportive, submissive wife. Later the regrets flourished: "Why didn't I have the courage to trust my own judgment when Lyall was determined to carry out his new ideas?"

I suppose he never made it easy for me. Whenever I objected to something I felt uneasy about, Lyall said, "Jean, you are disagreeing with me again. Are you doing this deliberately to oppose me? I know what I am doing. You're too negative and scared of your own shadow." I learned to be silent.

Now, when I look back, I realize Poppa wasn't an unreasonable man. He was mature enough to change his mind when I persisted or when I could demonstrate why it was important to investigate more thoroughly before moving forward. But I was a flight person. Like a coward, I backed down too easily. Hindsight tells me that when I knew I was right I should have raised more questions instead of backing down.

I don't believe I was a complementary or positive influence on Lyall when I acted like a doormat. I didn't truly honor him by backing down in fear. I was not being spiritual. I was neurotic in wanting to keep peace at any price. The times I did hold my ground, we both ended up reaping the rewards.

A few years ago, I sought some advice from Dr. Kirk Farnsworth, executive director of Crista Counseling Services. There were some areas of my life that were confusing, and I needed some objective counsel. One of the things he said to me during our time together was, "Jean, why do you doubt your own thinking so much? Trust your judgment. It is far better than you realize." How I wish someone had said that to me many years ago, when I was newly married, a young mother, and during those stressful years of raising teens. "Trust your judgment." That's good counsel. Grab it for yourself.

All of us have regrets; some have more than others. If you haven't yet experienced a time of recapitulation, you will. A story my father used to tell me as a child reminds me of my need to cling to God, especially during the more painful times of life.

Father was a great scholar, and he often talked of the Greek heroes of early literature. I could never hear enough about Ulysses, a king of ancient Greece who was compelled to embark on great adventures in search of knowledge.

Ulysses encountered countless perils on land and sea, but he and his brave sailors overcame every obstacle and persevered toward their goals at all cost. I found the courageous lives of these mythological heroes and heroines tremendously inspiring during my early years.

In my favorite story, Ulysses had grown old and wanted one last adventure before his death, so he chose a son to rule in his place, said farewell to his wife and peasants, and manned his ship with the bravest sailors in all of Greece. A few days into their travels he came upon a very narrow passage between treacherous rocky islands where the wicked Sirens lived. He knew the Sirens disguised themselves as beautiful maidens and that their singing had the power to lure innocent sailors ashore. Once the sailors were on land, the Sirens turned them into slaves or animals.

Ulysses knew his sailors wouldn't be able to resist the call of the Sirens, so he ordered his men to fill their ears with wax. Then he ordered them to lash him tightly to the main mast so he could not respond to the temptations of the seductive maidens. His ship sailed safely through the passageway, and the evil Sirens killed themselves in shame for failing to capture the ship.

I've traveled through treacherous waters, too, and needed to take precautions. Life has been unpredictable.

I don't know what kinds of tempests you are enduring right now, but I do know that God will do for you what He has done for me. If you ask Him, He will guide you through the storm, and when the air clears and the seas are calm, He'll be there, too, whether you feel you need Him or not. There is no mistake you have ever made, no injustice you have ever suffered, that can keep God from loving you. That's what His faithfulness is all about.

One of the places I have seen evidence of God's faithfulness in my life has been on the job. In the next chapter I'll show you some ways He has helped me endure dangerously high levels of job stress.

6

Job Stress

Job stress is mostly beyond our control, wherever we work. It comes with the paycheck. Although there is little we can do to eliminate it, there are ways to minimize its effects on us and discharge its tensions in a healthy, productive manner.

"Hello, Jean. You don't know me, but I know of you from several different people. My family is in deep trouble, and I need your services. Our teenage son has had several run-ins with the law, and now the juvenile judge says he must have professional counseling as part of his probation. The judge will not accept pastoral help for us anymore. I want to make an appointment with you immediately."

I sensed the desperation in her voice and knew my reply would be difficult for her to accept. "I am very sorry. I cannot schedule an appointment with you. I work for a large family agency with strict policies. Unless I am on intake duty when you call, you will be assigned to someone else. The agency doesn't allow clients to request specific counselors."

"That is ridiculous!" she said. "I was referred to you. I refuse to go to someone I don't know. Can't you see me privately?"

"I'm sorry. The agency rules don't allow private meetings such as you are suggesting. But the agency has many experienced therapists. I think a male counselor would be more helpful in your situation." I knew her son would need a strong male figure to help him work on his problems.

"Jean, can you guarantee another counselor who holds your same beliefs?"

I had to explain that it was against agency policy to discuss the therapist's personal beliefs.

"This is absurd!" she retorted. "I am worried sick about my son, and all you are giving me is stupid red tape!"

I voiced my confidence in the other therapists and urged her to call the agency for an appointment. A few weeks later I received a letter from this woman, warning me that if anything went wrong in their family, it would be my fault for not taking the case.

Six months later I was enjoying early morning tea while reading the *Seattle Times* and saw the headline: SEVENTEEN-YEAR-OLD SON STABS HIS MOTHER. I clutched the paper to my chest, groaning in disbelief, after reading that the victim was the woman I had turned away. Her son had stabbed her with a large kitchen knife when she refused to allow him to drive without a license.

The news spread like wildfire through the agency and was soon splashed across the pages of the *Seattle Times*. A therapist's nightmare came true when our case records were subpoenaed by the courts.

Living under this pressure was exhausting. I felt heavy anxiety twenty-four hours a day. The agency uproar had jeopardized my job, and I was the sole support of our family, since Lyall had unexpectedly lost his job in an organizational takeover. Two of our children were heading for medical training, and now my immediate supervisor was placing pressure on me to resign. With Seattle in a semi-recession and counseling jobs scarce, I knew I couldn't afford to resign.

I began living one moment at a time. There was little relief. Several times a day I whispered, "Lord, please help me."

In a most unexpected way, the Lord did intervene. The agency director, upon returning to the office after an illness, learned of the court hearings and was very affirming and supportive of me. He told another staff member, "Jean Lush was hired because of her outstanding influence in the Christian community. We need her in our agency. Before she started working with us, Christian clients didn't want to come here. Churches criticized us. We need to service people who have strong religious beliefs."

Then he briefed me on his plans for my future role in the agency. From then on, he wanted me to be available to church clients upon request.

The woman's son received years of expert counseling and supervision. Today he lives in another part of the United States with his wife and family. He has suffered deep remorse for what he did.

Why I Worked Outside Our Home

Women work outside the home for various legitimate reasons, but doing so is always stressful and requires a careful balancing of priorities.

It was winter. My car pool left the counseling center at 5:30 p.m., but I remained behind to counsel late into the evening. My assignment was to work nights and see clients who worked during regular office hours. At 9:00 p.m. I locked my office door and began the trek across the center of town to catch a bus traveling north to my suburb. The counseling center was located in the rough part of Seattle. I knew it wasn't safe walking the streets alone at night, but none of the buses came by the office, and I couldn't afford any other mode of transportation.

This went on week after week, month after month. I requested some relief from the agency, but no consideration was given to my request. I pleaded that I had done more nighttime work than anyone else, but my words fell on deaf ears. Oh, how I hated those nights in the winter!

In those days I was usually wound up and tense. Perhaps my anxieties were related to the fact that I was the first married woman in my family to ever work outside the home. My mother was a highly educated woman, but she never worked a day for pay after marriage. She did, however, accomplish many notable achievements within the community. Being a wife and mother who worked outside the home was not a script with which I was familiar.

I've had many young women ask me why I chose to work away from home. Actually, I don't have a simple answer, because I love being home. I first began work outside our home in full-time Christian ministry with Lyall. During those years I was also completing my graduate training as a therapist. I later worked full-time as a marriage and family therapist until I retired. In the early years, our family was financially destitute. I felt compelled to work so I could offer my children the opportunity to attend college.

Still, my drive wasn't based strictly on financial need. From the time I was a young adult, I felt God wanted to equip me to work with women. I followed His call.

Through the years, various opportunities came up that could have distracted me from this mission. I was offered a prestigious position with a large Christian radio station that wanted to expand its women's programs. During that same year I was also offered a full-time job with a large counseling agency that was staffed with seasoned psychologists and psychiatrists. The radio job sounded wonderful. All my friends encouraged me to expand my broadcasting skills and wondered why I would even think twice about the offer. My wise husband offered no suggestions either way. His comment was, "This is your world. You make the decision and then tell me what you want to do."

Some around me suggested, "Take the big radio job." One of my teenagers said, "Mom, all you want to do is grow roses and bake pies. This family needs more money and less mother. Go with the counseling job. It's full time." Having to make the decision sparked tension in me.

For some reason, the offer at the radio station didn't seem to be God's choice for me. I felt pulled toward the agency. I knew it was a coveted place to work and it would help me develop my clinical skills with women. It seemed to fit God's mission for me.

As it turned out, I accepted the job at the agency. There I spent a long period of my life learning how to counsel almost any family problem you can imagine. I also had the opportunity to do some specialized studies on the emotional phases of women. For years I led family-life groups for women between thirty-five and fifty-five. We studied the changing patterns of emotions in relation to fluctuating hormones. A wealth of wisdom came out of those years. Hindsight is 20/20, and now I know God helped me make the right decision.

In addition to God's leading, I can't underestimate the impact my family had on my decision to pursue a career.

Born into an intellectual home, I grew up feeling inferior to four of my family members who were brilliant high achievers. I wasn't like them. I learned slowly and had to be removed from school twice because of a strange nerve disease. Both times I had to repeat the grades I missed.

Ever since I can remember, I wanted to prove to my mother that I was someone she could admire. I'm certain that I was driven to complete graduate school and achieve professional status to prove to my parents that I was worthwhile. The last time I saw my mother, she said to me in passing, "You know, you really are quite bright." You will never know how deeply those words touched me. I was a grown woman with three older children, a booming clinical practice in Seattle, and regular guest appearances on radio talk shows, but as those words rolled off her tongue, I could think of nothing more important to me. I had finally arrived: I had won her approval. If you are a mother, let me remind you that it is never ever too late to encourage your children. It could change their lives.

I've mentioned three reasons why I worked outside my home. The decision is complex and tension-producing for many women, especially those with children. However, when young women do have a choice—an honest choice—I encourage them to stay home with their young children as much as possible, even if it means a financial loss.

Most surveys seem to agree that the primary reason women work is due to economic pressures. I have counseled hundreds of single mothers who yearned for the privilege of raising their children in a more wholesome fashion than what they were forced into by death or divorce. Few women I knew had the absolute freedom to choose whether they would or wouldn't work.

Job Stress among Women Is Universal

I recently read an international job survey that said 71 percent of women between thirty-five and forty-four work outside the home. The survey included 22,000 women from Asia, South America, Europe, and Australia. Fifty-five percent of American women who worked claimed that they would work even if they were not pressured by financial reasons.[1]

I found it interesting that 39 percent of the women in this survey rated their jobs as very stressful, and another 55 percent said their jobs were somewhat stressful. The sources of highest job stress were the inability to control the work pace and problems from home spilling over into work. Newspapers report that women complain of job stress related to abrupt changes, pay inequity, overwork, and sexual harassment. Of course all this causes fatigue. At the same time, the mental health field is reporting higher rates of depression among women, who are two times more likely than men to suffer bouts of major depression. I cannot help but think that the higher numbers of working women and increased percentage of depression among women are somehow related.

I've always been interested in both male and female perspectives on women in the workplace. Throughout my career, I frequently spoke to junior- and senior-high students at public high schools. When I asked the boys to tell me what they thought about working wives, the answers fifteen years ago were radically different from the ones I heard more recently. Today's students say, "Of course wives have to work, at least for the first few years of marriage. How on earth could we get a good start, otherwise?" Fifteen years ago, very few boys publicly admitted they wanted their wives to contribute to the family income. Times have changed. I noticed in my counseling practice that men who married a second time seemed very impressed with successful working women.

Job stress is a fact of life that will continue as long as we are working. This is true whether our job is in or out of our home, or a combination of the two. We must learn to take good care of ourselves and buffer stress, so we can keep plodding forward and not burn out halfway through the race. I've asked hundreds of men and women what they do to reduce the negative effects of job stress. Here is a condensed list of suggestions they've offered.

I Lower My Job Stress By:

- Consistent exercise
- Eight to nine hours of sleep each night
- Weekly recreation
- Weekend activities that are a complete contrast to my work
- Guarding one day a week for rest and worship
- Taking intermittent days off during high-pressure seasons
- Saying no and not feeling guilty
- Tending to my personal needs
- Restructuring priorities
- Eating a nutritious breakfast with an added protein drink
- Annual vacations
- Accepting a job that offers less pay but more satisfaction
- Working one day a week less
- Refusing to become obsessed with my job

- Pretending my job doesn't exist when I'm not there
- Leaving my work at the office
- Developing empathy for my associates
- Striving for team spirit on the job
- Sharing stresses with other women at work
- Giving myself some perks such as lunch out with the girls
- Making allowances for my supervisor's stresses
- Turning a deaf ear to office gossip
- Committing each day to God and thanking Him for little things
- Treating myself gently when I make mistakes
- Closing my eyes, taking deep breaths, and asking God to fill me with His peace

Through the years I've probably used every one of these ideas many times. They were like cool drinks on a scorching-hot day; they didn't magically make the heat disappear, but they did offer me a soothing bit of relief and gave me the boost I needed to deal with job-related stress.

7

Unmet Needs

No one's life is perfect, and none of us feel that all our needs are being met. Sometimes we actually feel deprived because of this, and deprivation leads to tension.

A woman who seemed to have everything going for her requested counseling from me. She said she was very unhappy and wanted to explore the possibility of a divorce. I was a bit puzzled by her request, because she had financial security, everything she wanted for her home and children, and a loyal, faithful husband. Yet she described herself as very unhappy because her husband did not meet her needs.

I said to her, "May I ask you a question?" With her nod of approval, I continued. "Suppose your husband was in a sudden accident that left him crippled for life. Knowing that he couldn't meet your physical needs the way he does now, how would you manage? What would you do?"

"Oh, there wouldn't be any question as to what I would do," she said. "It would be my duty to stay with him and do what I could for him."

"You mean if he were incapable of looking after you and meeting your needs you'd feel different about the idea of divorce?" I pressed.

"Well, yes," she said. "I would feel different."

"Can you tell me why?" I continued, wondering what I would hear next.

"Well," she said, "I'd feel different because I would know that he couldn't possibly meet my needs."

Her answer was just what I needed to drive home my point.

"I'm telling you right now that your husband cannot possibly meet all your emotional and romantic needs. He's handicapped."

I had seen her husband. He was the tall, gorgeous, outdoor type: hardworking, dedicated, sturdy, strong, somewhat stoic.

"Look at it this way," I went on. "Your husband is emotionally handicapped to meet all your needs. He's just not wired for it. I'd say 90 percent of the men alive on this planet are not equipped to handle all of a woman's emotional needs. Much of their conditioning doesn't allow this to happen. Their primary role as provider drains their emotional and psychic energy, leaving little remaining for fulfilling romantic needs."

I could almost read her thoughts: *But the savvy men of today are tender and romantic.* I continued, "Soap operas and romance novels give us the idea that we must live for love. Have you ever wondered when the guys on those soaps work? They spend hours home during lunch, displaying a marvelous understanding of the soulish nature of women. I think Hollywood is doing a good job of making women feel they are married to someone who is below par."

Our conversation continued as the clock ticked past the hour, and by the close of our session this young lady had some things to contemplate. We spent several hours together in following weeks, sorting through her feelings and examining her expectations. It wasn't long before she began to feel better about herself and her marriage, largely due to her change in perspective.

I'm Lonely

June was immaculately dressed, drove an expensive car, and lived in an affluent neighborhood. Just after her thirtieth birthday, she came in to talk with me.

Her husband, Mark, worked with his father in a prospering business and was soon to inherit the company. He worked long hours in management, learning everything he could to get a firm grip on the operations. With his father's retirement near, he wanted to be well prepared to handle the responsibilities alone. Outside competition was intense, as there were several other growing companies trying to break into his market.

June came to me depressed, suffering with headaches, and complaining that her husband did not meet her emotional needs.

"I don't understand why I feel so awful," June lamented. "Mark is a wonderful provider. He's given me more than I ever had growing up. I always dreamed about living in a house like ours. But I'm lonely. Mark is always working. I'd rather live in a tent with a man who understands my feelings than in the palace I have now."

She spoke of a relationship she once had with a musician whom she nearly married. He was very romantic, and seemed to understand her. She loved him but knew he could never provide the material security that was extremely important to her. She had grown up deprived and was determined never to return to that way of life.

Now she doubted her decision. She wanted love and attention. She suffered terribly with premenstrual tension, and during certain times of the month felt she was going crazy. I knew firsthand what she meant. During these frightening times, she craved her husband's emotional embrace.

When I met Mark, I found him to be deeply committed to his beautiful wife. He appreciated her homemaking skills and credited her with the beauty of their home. He also admitted that most of his time and energy was spent on the business. There were a couple of reasons for this—his father's pending retirement and his wife's expensive tastes. Apparently she had a great love of original oil paintings. Their home was filled with them, and each piece cost a small fortune.

As I contemplated their case, I realized June's romantic expectations of marriage would never be met, because no ordinary man could ever fill the bottomless well inside her. I tried to explain my perspective to her.

"June, there is a little nugget that has helped me over the years in my own marriage. Men and women are born and raised on different planets. Men are a little strange; women are a little weird. Men are taught to express tenderness with caution, for fear it may be misconstrued as weakness and hinder their competitive edge in the world. They find their adult male maturity in the arena of their vocations. Since their work is who they are, they must be tough-minded and strong in order to survive.

"Women, on the other hand, are raised to be tender, emotional, and nurturing. In subtle ways they are conditioned to find a Prince Charming who will romantically love them all the days of their lives. Most women get the impression that there is only one man in the world who is destined to be their perfect mate.

"The tragedy is that many young women judge their marriage solely on whether their husband is able to make them feel romantic. They may have a good marriage that will help them achieve their highest potential, but feel deprived because their romantic needs aren't satisfied."

June had chosen a husband who met her dominant needs far better than she realized at the time. Her desire for security and a beautiful home were basic to her happiness. It was unfortunate she had lingering romantic illusions about the restless musician who wanted her to share his wandering adventures and his poverty. The stark reality of that life would have destroyed her romantic feelings very quickly, but she didn't realize this, and her musician friend became her ghost lover.

Marriage counselors are well aware that many women develop ghost lovers. This may be somebody they knew in the past or someone who appears in their dreams, in a book, or on television. The ghost lover may even be somebody they know. Some women, disappointed about their unmet needs in marriage, return to a fantasyland with a ghost lover. Some counselors think this is fine. In my opinion it's a waste of time and creates more problems than it's worth. I believe the Lord can meet our emotional needs much more effectively than a ghost lover. We need to turn to Him when we feel a void in our soul, not to some conjured-up fantasy.

Ten years later, I ran into June at a local mall. At the time she had two children in grade school and was grateful for her faithful husband and the security he provided. I don't think he had changed much, but she was happier because her expectations about romance had changed.

When I was writing my first book, *Emotional Phases of a Woman's Life*, I decided to investigate the reading material women were buying. I called bookstores and secondhand shops that handled thousands of paperbacks. One morning, in a used-book store, I witnessed a woman bringing in a huge sack of romantic novels to exchange for dozens more. I asked her why she read so many of these books, and she said, "I love romance. It's my escape from a humdrum life, I guess."

I also wrote publishers, requesting specific information about romantic novel sales. Harlequin Publishers sent some facts and figures that were surprising to me. In 1984 they sold over 200 million paperbacks. I'm sure the number is larger today. A survey conducted by Zondervan Publishers showed that 52 percent of the women polled bought romantic novels regularly. Other bookstores reported that some customers binge buy these books.

Why is there such a colossal market for romantic paperbacks? Some would say this is one positive way women can stimulate their love life. However, many romance novel readers admit to being addicted to these books. They express a desire to break the habit because it robs them of time for other healthy involvements.

I think these books serve as a substitute for reality for some women who do not feel romantically fulfilled, but I question the benefits of getting lost in fiction. If anything, this habit may stir up unrealistic expectations and make them feel less satisfied with life as it is.

Making Him More Romantic

I am often asked, "How can I encourage my husband to be more romantic?" I'll share an incident from my life that might help answer the question. When I was married to

Lyall, I knew that if I tried to demand more romance, the romance we did have would be quickly squelched. So I tried some other approaches.

On our last wedding anniversary, I knew Lyall wasn't making plans for a celebration, so rather than brood, I decided to make some special lunch arrangements and be excited anyway. I bought an expensive book about Monet and his famous garden in France. Then I called a beautiful waterfront restaurant with a marvelous view of the Edmond ferries and made a reservation for two. This was one of Lyall's favorite places to dine.

We had a leisurely lunch, ordering our favorite crab cakes and a gourmet dessert. When we got home, Poppa's gift and a love letter full of my appreciation for him was waiting for him on the dining room table. Late in the evening we shared a romantic little supper. I made his favorite fruit salad filled with tropical specialty fruits.

I still laugh when I think about that day. Lyall was caught completely off guard. All the festivities confused him because he had forgotten our anniversary, but once he figured out what was going on, he tried to pretend he was prepared. He made a quiet phone call to the florist, only to find that they couldn't deliver on such short notice. Finally, he admitted that he had forgotten our anniversary. The funny part was his uneasiness over my enjoyment of the occasion in spite of his memory lapse. He never forgot that day because I was so animated and charming and never said anything about his forgetting to make the day special for me.

The day after our anniversary, Lyall called our daughter and asked her to remind him of birthdays and anniversaries ahead of time. The following Christmas, he was prepared. He went to our favorite department store and asked a saleslady he recognized which perfume I liked best. With her help, he had a gift package containing my favorite fragrance especially made for me. You should have seen him Christmas morning. He triumphantly presented me with his gift, grinning from ear to ear.

Perhaps you're thinking that Lyall didn't care enough to bother before, but that wasn't the case. He was the ninth child born on a sheep station in Australia. He had a wonderful childhood, but his family gave low priority to birthdays and anniversaries.

I remember something I learned in my clinical studies that applies here. My professors taught me about the law of repetition compulsion: that which happened to us in our family of origin, we will cause to happen in our present family.

When women ask me, "How can I change my husband? How can I get him to meet my needs?" I have to say, "It's not easy, because he was very well-conditioned before he ever met you. More romance from him may well depend on your choice to accept and treasure him *as he is*. If he doesn't sense acceptance and feels you are pushing him to change, he may simply become more resistant. He needs to feel loved as he is. When this is firmly established, then changes may come slowly."

I also believe that too much discussion about unmet needs in a marriage can rob romance of its mystique. Treat romance as you would a delicate and beautiful flower that can be scorched by the hot sun (quarreling and harsh words) or withered by frost (coldness and indifference). Like a beautiful flower, romance must be nurtured, fertilized, and watered on a regular basis. Then the blooming will come naturally.

A Shift in Focus

Recently I was invited to speak at a large women's retreat. My younger daughter, Heather, loves to travel with me. Sometimes when we are at conferences she acts as if she doesn't know me and sits in the middle of the audience, listening for audience reactions as I speak.

At this particular conference she sat beside a highly educated middle-aged woman who was a leader in her church. At the end of one of the meetings, the woman said, "That lady has changed my life. For the last forty years I've held a grudge against my husband because I've felt cheated out of romance. For years I've dreamed about meeting a special man who would fulfill my greatest fantasies. I have a wonderful family, but I've always yearned for something more. Today I'm letting go of that grudge. I want to tell my husband how grateful I am for his faithfulness to me and the great role model he is for our three sons. That lady will never know how much her talk has meant to me."

With a smile, Heather replied, "Yes, she will. She's my mother, and she'll love hearing your story on our way home."

Hearing this lady's reaction reminded me of another woman I knew many years before who found an answer to her unmet needs. I met Mrs. Hastings during my university years.

While attending an Easter conference for university students, I heard for the first time why Jesus Christ had come to earth, and that He wanted to be my personal Savior and friend. I approached the conference leader after the meeting and said, "I want Jesus Christ to be my personal Savior and Lord." Right then I prayed quietly and asked God to forgive my sins and take charge of my life. My overall physical and emotional health dramatically changed. For the first time in my life, I was spiritually alive.

Following my conversion I was hungry to learn all I could about the Bible. I attended an Inter-Varsity Christian

Fellowship meeting regularly at Holy Trinity Church and sought out other teachers, too. That's how I met Mrs. Hastings. She invited me and some of my friends to a weekly Bible study in her home. I studied with her for twelve months. At the close of the school year, I asked her to share her life story with me.

"Well, Jean, I was born in an old shipping port town in England. We lived there for many years, and sometime during my early childhood I asked God to forgive my sins and to come into my heart. Our family went to the local Methodist church in town. I can still remember that old preacher's evangelistic flair.

"As a young teenager I was part of a preaching band. We held meetings in the streets and most anywhere we could draw a crowd, weather permitting. Sailors wandering the streets at night with little to do gathered to hear us sing and share our stories about God's work in our lives.

"One night a tall, good-looking young man asked to talk with me after hearing me speak. I invited him to our church, and he asked God to take control of his life. He was passionate about learning the Bible, and in time he eventually became the leader of our preaching group.

"He was a dynamic young man. I have to admit I was very attracted to him, but the attraction was mutual. We worked together in the preaching band for several years. The more time we spent together, the deeper my love grew for him. Jack had stolen my heart.

"I knew Jack was destined for something extraordinary. We talked about sharing the rest of our lives together, but realized that we couldn't set a wedding date until we knew this was what God wanted for both of us. We each vowed to seek God's counsel and to obey Him. It was obvious to me that God's blessing was on our relationship. We were very effective, ministering together.

"As it turned out, we decided to apply to our Methodist Overseas Missionary Board for consideration as missionaries. The board interviewed both of us, and Jack was immediately accepted. I was turned down with no explanation. It was hard for me to understand, since I had been active in Christian evangelism for many years, but I didn't question what was happening.

"Jack soon left town and joined his fellow missionary candidates for training in South Africa. We were avid writers. I loved reading his letters, always believing that somehow, someday, we would be married. I was certain a love as deep as ours could never be parted.

"Then one afternoon Father asked me to sit with him in the parlor. He didn't do this often, so I knew he wanted to talk about something important. I'll never forget his words: 'Marian, you must give up all hope of a future with Jack.'

"He went on to tell me that the missionary board had selected six young volunteers who were willing to give up all their home ties to venture into the heart of the Congo. Jack had volunteered. I knew I would never be able to join him, because the Belgian government forbid women from entering the dangerous wilds of the Congo. There was a good chance Jack would never return alive.

"I cried for weeks—no, years. My parents were very concerned about my blue moods and talked with our pastor. His remedy was simple. He would find me another fine young Christian man in the church who would be a suitable husband.

"So I married George, and we emigrated to Australia to begin a new life together. But the aching for Jack never went away. I couldn't forget him. I felt like I was living a double life, never telling anyone how I really felt inside. George knew about my broken engagement to Jack, but never guessed it still bothered me. He probably thought I was fulfilled and happy to have a home and two beautiful daughters.

"One morning I awoke at dawn to read my Bible and pray, but I couldn't see the words on the page through my tears. I felt like I was mentally 'cracking up.' I fell on my face, begging God to help me.

"Jean, God visited me that morning. I don't know what to call the experience, but God touched me in a supernatural way. He let me know in my heart that He had heard my cries, and He had a mission for my life. I was to dedicate myself to studying the Bible, because He was going to use me to teach the Scriptures. It seemed a bit odd to me, because the only people I knew who taught Scripture were men. But, I believed what He said."

Mrs. Hastings had heard from God, and this dear lady held Bible classes in her home until she retired to a rest home. Single-handedly she was responsible for teaching and equipping thirty-three young men and women who went on to become seasoned missionaries. In those days, there was no such thing as a Bible college. She was it.

As a young woman, hoping to someday marry, I felt sad she had lost Jack to the Congo. I asked her if she regretted not being able to share her life with the man she so dearly loved. Her response rather startled me. "My dear, I would not have it otherwise," she said firmly. "If I had married Jack, I would have been his slave, and never would have matured. Today, I *know* my Lord Jesus in a way I never could have, had I married Jack. No, I have no regrets."

Unmet needs and tension are traveling companions. Sometimes our needs can be satisfied through natural means, other times the supernatural touch of God is required.

What are your needs? How do you need God to intervene for you? Talk with Him about your sources of tension. Ask Him for wisdom and guidance. Ask Him for answers. God is not partial. He will do for you what He has done for me and Susan, June, Mrs. Hastings, and countless others. His ears will hear your cry, and He will act on your behalf, but it all must start with you. Carve out some time to be alone with Him. Tune your ears to listen to His Spirit. Open your heart to receive from Him. Then get ready. Watch. Wait. In time, you'll sense Him filling the holes in your soul.

Over fifty years have passed since Mrs. Hastings told me her story, but her words still ring in my ears: "I have no regrets." Few people can make that statement. Mrs. Hastings said it with conviction. Perhaps that's the result of daily seeking God and obeying His voice, whatever the cost.

8

Parenting Pressures

Anyone who has children knows that parenting can be stressful. Children fight, disobey, and insist on being themselves—all of which can drive parents crazy with worry and tension. How can we deal with this type of tension in our lives?[1]

Sibling Rivalry

Dan and Robert are brothers who are less than one year apart. Dan was born to a teenage mother and adopted at birth by Susan. A few months after the adoption, Susan conceived, and nine months later, she gave birth to Robert. Two years later, her beautiful daughter, Marie, was born. This little girl had the sunniest disposition of any child I've known. Wherever she went, people fell in love with her. A few years later, Susan became a single mother after a tragic divorce.

Though the two boys are close in age, they are very different. Dan is mechanically inclined, and his possessions are important to him. When he is aggravated, he explodes and acts out his anger in physical ways. Robert, however, is articulate and uses teasing as his deadly weapon. Poor Susan has her hands full.

What's the answer? First of all, I think it helps mothers to know that sibling rivalry is normal. Quarreling is to be expected and is sometimes useful, since the stresses children go through with their siblings may give them resources they can use later in life.

There are siblings who don't fight. I don't think we can assume that this is strictly the product of skilled parenting, because many skilled parents have children who quarrel. Sometimes a family simply has quiet children who avoid conflict. There are also cases where violent parents produce children who are terrified of any form of trouble. The motto these children live by is "Peace at all costs."

Dr. James Dobson says that when women are asked, "What is the most irritating part of raising children?" the unanimous answer is, "Sibling rivalry!" Most parents are deeply concerned about the bickering they hear between their kids. A great deal of energy goes into settling battles and trying to teach children to get along together. However, in most households, no amount of preaching will entirely solve the problem. Parents can lower their own anxieties by dropping the belief that good homes don't have quarrels. Show me a "good family," and I'll bet we'll find children who have their moments of war!

Some experts say that parents should stay completely out of their children's quarrels. Perhaps this works at times, but I'm not sure I agree with the concept across the board. When small and large children are involved in a squabble, there is good reason for a mother to mediate. The younger child doesn't have the strength of the older one and needs protection. Mothers who have children of varying ages at home need to be "all ears."

Quarreling usually doesn't happen without reason. There are definite purposes behind it. Every fight has three layers: the immediate cause of trouble; the struggle for status; and the underlying core of resentment built up from years of rivalry for possession of the parent.[2]

We see this in Dan and Robert's rivalry. When Robert took one of Dan's toys from his room, there was an immediate cause for trouble. As the two of them fought, each struggled to show who was in control and most powerful. Dan attacked physically; Robert used verbal barbs. Of course, all this was within Susan's hearing. As soon as the fight began, they knew her attention was hooked.

Susan was usually wise to these tactics and let the boys settle matters between themselves. This was a good approach, since they were so close in age. In most respects they were an even match for each other. By not rushing to the scene whenever they fought, she didn't reward the behavior she wanted stopped. Dan and Robert learned they couldn't get their mom's undivided attention by squabbling.

Some Siblings Don't Like Each Other

If children chronically quarrel, why have them play together? Why give them the chance to fight? Why not separate them? I've posed these ideas to mothers before, only to hear, "That's ridiculous. They're brothers, and they must get along."

The truth is that some siblings don't like each other. Maybe they have completely different interests or personalities. Just being in the presence of one may irritate the other. This is horrifying to an idealistic mother who thinks it's her job to make her kids love one another. She feels like a failure or that her Christian image is tarnished because her children fight.

Just because children are siblings doesn't mean they will automatically be good friends. It helps to keep a long-range view in mind. Sibling relationships tend to get better as time passes.

It's Okay to Have Bad Feelings

Children can be taught it's normal to have good and bad feelings toward family members. Encouraging siblings to tell each other when they are mad or happy may improve communication and prevent silent wars from lingering for days. Nonetheless, this kind of openness doesn't happen overnight. Many children find it difficult to discuss angry feelings. Their guilt over anger ties their tongues. Parents must give children the right to talk about these unpleasant feelings and then consistently encourage them to do so.

A boy who lives in the shadow of achieving brothers and sisters often does not feel good about himself. He may tend to provoke other siblings because it gives him a sense of superiority. He may not be as smart, athletic, or good-looking as his brothers and sisters, but he can control his "enemies" by making them upset.

Parents are naturally drawn to self-assured children who have pleasant dispositions; but the less-confident, troubled child needs more of his parents' time. If he feels appreciated and loved, he'll be less likely to clamor for attention. Individual time alone with a parent can help him feel secure so he doesn't have to try to one-up his brothers and sisters. A forty-five minute weekly date with Mom or Dad can work wonders.

If children are having extreme difficulties tolerating one another, parents may need to explain the difference between actions and feelings. They can insist that children act respectfully toward one another regardless of their feelings. If a child acts unkindly by hitting, swearing, or name-calling, he should be required to apologize for his poor behavior. He must be responsible for his actions, whether his feelings change or not.

This can be taken one step further. You have heard the saying "Feelings follow actions." When we go out of our way to be kind to someone we don't like, our feelings tend to change in the process. At family gatherings, children can be prompted to share positive things they see or like about one another. This will help them appreciate the uniqueness of each individual.

Disrespect or a Healthy Expression of Feelings?

When I was talking with a teenager today I asked, "What makes you most angry with grown-ups?" Without hesitating she answered, "I hate it when my parents say, 'Don't talk back!' I hate it when they yell at me before I can tell my side of the story. I think I should have a chance to explain things, even when I'm wrong."

I asked her to help me understand what she meant. She said, "Like today. I came home from school and said I wanted a snack. Mom said, 'No, you can't, because you are always overeating!' She was ticked-off before I walked in the door, and dumped it on me. Later in the afternoon Mom yelled from the kitchen, 'Elizabeth, come here right now.'

"I called back, 'I can't, I'm right in the middle of an algebra problem and it's important I finish it.'

"Then she blew the roof off, screaming, 'You come down here this minute and don't you dare talk back to me.' Twenty minutes later she harped at me for not getting better grades in math. I wish my parents were as consistent as my teachers."

Maybe you're thinking Elizabeth acts too big for her britches. Actually, she's not a sassy child. She is responsible, attractive, and a bright, rational fourteen-year-old. It bothers her that her parents overreact and aren't more sensitive.

I was curious to hear more, so I asked Elizabeth what she did when she was angry with her parents.

"I go to my room and yell and kick and jump up and down. Sometimes I bury my head in my pillow and cry. When I calm down, I write in my diary."

I'm going to raise a question as an active grandparent: What can we do to protect our children from stuffing their feelings, and yet not allow them to be defiant or disrespect-ful? How can we guard ourselves from forcing them to shut down their emotions and at the same time teach them self-control and respect for authority? We can't allow them to fling their anger at us whenever we oppose them, or they'll never fare well in the real world, but is it beneficial to forbid all expressions of anger?

When we want to teach our children how to manage their anger, we must start by examining ourselves. We are our children's role models. They will unconsciously absorb the way we act when we are angry. Perhaps the way they act is a reflection of the way we act with them. I know many mothers say things such as, "Don't you dare display that kind of anger in this home." Sometimes strong-willed children argue, "Why not? You do it all the time!" or "You and Daddy argue all the time. What's the big deal?"

It is useless to say, "I am an adult, and you are a child. I can do things you can't," or "Do as I say, not as I do." The child of today would say his parent doesn't make sense, and he'd be right.

If our lives are inconsistent with what we teach, our children will not give us a position of authority in their lives. They'll rationalize their temper, saying, "I can't help getting so mad. It's just the way I am. Like father, like son." If a child lives with others who consistently lose their temper, tantrums become the norm rather than the exception. We must ask ourselves: Do we swallow our negative feelings or use them to verbally assault those around us? What are our children intuitively catching from us? Are we teaching our children how to manage their anger, or is their anger managing us and them?

Three cousins who were eight, nine, and ten stayed in my home one summer. They decided they wanted to walk to a shopping mall two miles away, and they wanted to go alone. I happened to know that the movie theater at the mall was a prime hangout for drug peddlers.

I was nervous about their idea and answered their request with a no. They gave me the usual arguments: "You don't trust us. How come you let the boys go places by themselves? We can look after ourselves. We never get to do anything around here. You're mean!"

After they complained several minutes, I turned to them and said, "I mean no."

This infuriated them even more, and they started in on me again. I switched the focus of their anger from me to their feelings of anger. I said, "Look, I understand that you are very angry with me. I would be feeling the same way if I were in your place. I know you think I am unfair, unreasonable, and downright mean. I know I am hard on you, and it must be awful for you to have a grandmother who is protective. By the way, Poppa wants to take you for a ferry ride as soon as he is finished in the studio."

Once again I resumed my defense. "If I were your age, I would feel exactly like you. I would be very angry and totally frustrated. But I would never say what you said to me. I have allowed all of you to tell me how you feel. I have listened. But now I want you to know that I've heard enough. No matter what you say, you will not change my answer. I know how you go on and on with your mothers, wearing them down until they let you do what you want. It won't work with me." With a slight smirk on my face, I finished the conversation by saying, "You've been at my house enough times to know I am a witch. Look at me. These are the steely blue eyes of a British witch, but I love you too much to give in."

When an important issue concerns the well-being of our children, it is extremely important that we don't back down from our original stand. Children quickly learn if a display of anger gets them what they want. If we give in to their pleading or fits, we condition them to use anger to their advantage. The next thing we know, they're doing this at school, too.

We've all seen an angry toddler in a shopping cart at the supermarket. As his mother wheels him up and down the aisles, the child demands one thing after another. When he doesn't get his way, he howls and kicks as though he were being terribly abused. This is humiliating for the tired mother who sees the looks that say: "Why doesn't she keep that kid under control?"

If this mother gives in, she loses the battle and her two-year-old learns exactly how to get what he wants. So what should she do? Never give in. Ignore this tantrum and keep telling him you aren't going to change your mind. If you need to, cut the outing short. If he enjoys going to the supermarket, tell him that next time he will not be allowed to go with you. The child must learn that his temper will not meet his needs.

Years ago my four-year-old granddaughter came back from overseas, where she had been living for eighteen months. She had a hard time coping with the many changes and refused to eat American food. She didn't sleep well and was angry with her mother, blaming her for all the changes.

After she had been with us for a short time, we took her and her family to visit one of her cousins who lived 150 miles away. When we pulled onto the freeway, this four-year-old suddenly started throwing a tantrum. She kicked and screamed bloody murder. We all warned her that Lyall could not drive on the freeway when she was screaming and she must stop. The tantrum continued. Lyall pulled off the road in a precarious place and I picked her up, still kicking and screaming, and climbed through a fence into a field. Holding her firmly, I said, "You must stop. We are not going home until you do." She yelled louder. Finally I said, "Poppa and your mother are very upset, and your mother is crying. I am going to pray for you louder than you can scream."

The scene was funny. There we were, on the side of the road, loudly competing with each other. Cars slowed down to see what was going on. She finally calmed down, and we got back in the car, but peace didn't last. As soon as we got back onto the freeway, she started screaming, "I hate you! And I hate my mother!" Lyall pulled over again, and we waited it out. I said, "We may be here all night, but you are not going to kick and scream in this car." This time she sensed we had the upper hand, and she calmed down. It never happened again. Today she is a splendid college student who feels very good about herself. By the way, she also learned the art of self-control very well.

Mothers and fathers need not be afraid of allowing their children to express negative feelings, even when those feelings are directed toward the parent. I think more damage is done to a child's emotional health when he or she is taught that anger is bad and sinful. My general rule is freedom within limits, but the parent is the one to determine the degree of freedom and set the limits.

Limits are important. If a child threatens a parent, the child has crossed a line. "I hate you, and I hope you die," can be calmly responded to with, "I know you are angry with me, and I understand why you are angry, but I won't take that kind of talk from anybody. You may go to your room this minute!" If a child screams, "I'll kill you," or "I'll kill myself," I suggest the parent consult a pediatrician or competent child therapist.

The Family Conference

Many years ago, when Lyall and I were in charge of a large girls' dormitory, a crisis occurred. It was a school rule that all the girls were to report back to me at midnight after social gatherings. The girls were also not allowed to leave the campus after a big weekend celebration unless their parents escorted them home. The rules were necessary for obvious reasons.

The older girls who lived in the dorm were furious because the day students didn't have to abide by the same rules. The seniors demanded a showdown with me.

I said, "Girls, suppose I told you right now that the rules were changed and you could come and go as you like, whenever you like? Would you want your younger sisters in this dormitory to have these freedoms?"

Silence. Most of them had younger sisters. "No! Of course not. They couldn't handle the freedom. They need to be supervised at all times."

The girls instantly backed down and said they would co-operate. This seemed too easy to me, and I was worried they were just playing up to me. Would they really obey the rules? These girls were seventeen and eighteen years old; there really wasn't much I could do to stop them from disobeying. I was amazed. After the confrontation in my quarters, the girls took pride in checking in before the clock chimed midnight.

Sometimes holding a family conference to talk about things that make us angry can be very helpful. We do ourselves and our children a favor when we allow open discussion about frustrations. When we encourage everyone in the family to participate in the discussion, children learn that anger is a natural part of life and it's okay to talk about our feelings.

When parents hold family conferences, they must listen quietly and carefully, with their hearts as well as their minds. When children are angry at a parent, it can help to ask, "If you were in my place right now, and you had a little boy or a little girl, what would you do?"

Some Children Are Contentious

Over the years I've noticed that certain children are by nature more argumentative and find enjoyment in picking fights. This happens especially when they're bored and have nothing better to do. My son, David, was an expert at this. He specialized in teasing his sisters and knew exactly how to provoke them. The rewards were wonderful for him: The girls became furious and exploded. He gloated over his victims and then innocently asked, "How did I know she would get so mad over nothing?" He was skillful in provoking me, too.

Some children are more contentious from birth. Naturally these children demand and need more of our time and attention. When a child continually overreacts in anger, set aside more time to be with him. Schedule one special date a week for you and your child. Go out for an ice-cream cone, take a walk, or do something the child especially enjoys. The goal of the outing is closeness and fun. Look at it as a chance to encourage your child with loving words and your undivided attention, not a time for focusing on his or her problems.

Leave room in your schedule for more interaction at bedtime. Storytelling is important because it makes the child feel special. Children love to hear stories about their parents' childhood, games they played, places they went, and some of their favorite memories. Sometimes it helps them to hear about the hardships and painful experiences their parents endured. This lets them know Mom and Dad are real people who felt joy, sorrow, and anger during childhood.

Children have an inner radar that detects if their parents are relaxed and focused on them. If they sense love and attention, they are more likely to share their troubles and fears. Heather taught me this when she was nine.[3]

At the time, Lyall and I lived in a girls' dormitory. He taught in the high school, and I was in charge of the girls in the dorm. One winter night the principal of the school warned me to be on guard around the clock, because he had heard a rumor that some of the younger girls were planning to sneak out of the dorm. I was jittery all evening and watched closely for anything unusual.

I suddenly noticed it was 8:30 p.m., the time I always spent with Heather. We had a bedtime ritual that was very important to her. During the daytime, it was difficult for me to have private time with Heather because I had to "mother" numerous other youngsters as well as my own. So every evening we had our own special time together.

I rushed down to find Heather. She was unusually slow and quiet that night. I was the opposite, frantically busy and tense. I kept trying to think of a way to settle her into bed in less time than usual.

The minutes ticked by and Heather did not budge from her slow pace despite my direct hints. "I don't have much time tonight, Heather, you will have to hurry." She ignored my words and signals. My feelings began to boil. At last she climbed into bed and asked me to tuck her in. Then she fussed because the covers were not quite straight.

I stood up, hoping to avoid further conversation, my ears alert for any unusual noises coming from the main area of the dormitory. I was about to hurry away when she said, "Mom. Sit down on my bed and talk to me." I sat on the bed, rigid and anxiously poised for flight, still listening for sounds from the dormitory.

"Mommy. I want to talk to you."

"What is it, dear?" I replied.

"I can't talk to you when you are *like that*!"

I tried to relax, and then said, "Come on, dear, what do you want to say to me?" I was hoping there wasn't anything important to discuss, because I needed to get back to the main dormitory.

"Please lie down with me on my bed," Heather said.

"Oh, all right." Heather was absolutely silent after I lay down, and I was getting very impatient. "If you want to tell me something, Heather, go ahead. Tell me about it now."

I'll never forget what she said after that: "Mommy, I can't talk to you the way you are tonight. You must *lie down in your soul first*."

At that point I threw thoughts of the dormitory out of my head and gave Heather my undivided attention. My body went limp. Heather obviously felt the difference, because after that she unloaded the tremendous burden she had been carrying all day.

"All the kids in class tease me because I lisp. Today the teacher made fun of me by imitating the way I talk in front of the whole class. Then she said I talked like that because I like being a baby."

The tears flowed. Heather had been completely humiliated. Then she cried out, "Why didn't you and Daddy tell me I sounded awful? Why didn't you do something about it? The teacher said I have a problem." I assured her the problem would be handled the next morning.

I went straight to the principal, who specialized in helping children with speech problems. He gladly gave Heather therapy, and the lisp was corrected in time.

I learned a big lesson from this incident. Children are very sensitive to the way we respond to them. We cannot fool our kids about the quality of our attentiveness. The moral of the story is, your children need to *feel* heard. When you listen, lie down in your soul first.

What Should I Do?

I'd like to close this chapter with some basic dos and don'ts for parents who are worn out by their children's angry outbursts. No one has a magic answer to this problem, but here is a summary of ideas that are known to help:

Please Don't

- feel guilty and condemn yourself
- make the oldest child responsible for keeping his anger in check all the time
- lash back at a child who is exploding

- condemn your child for feeling angry
- expect your child to put a smile on his face when he is angry
- pretend nothing is wrong when your child is angry
- jump right in and punish a child for being angry without knowing the whole story
- reward tantrums by giving in
- set your child up for an explosion by provoking him

Please Do

- listen to your children when they are angry
- give your children permission to feel anger without guilt
- set limits on how long your children can vent their anger
- tell your children that they have a right to feel angry but must never harm anyone or anything when they are angry
- arrange for an angry child to spend some time alone to cool down and think about what caused the outburst
- spend time with a child who has lashed out after he has cooled down
- teach children that anger is a natural part of life
- teach children several options they can use to diffuse their anger
- teach children how to forgive
- pray with your children about their feelings in a positive, understanding way
- hold your children close after they have cooled down. Many youngsters are terrified by their own anger.[4]

If I were to sum up my thoughts in this chapter, I'd say, Mom and Dad, hang in there. Time has a way of dulling swords. I know many children who screamed and yelled at their parents and siblings as youngsters, and they are good friends today. Then again, others still flare up with little reason, but they are more capable of putting on their best behavior in front of others. In either case, life gets more pleasant as they get older—even if older means after twenty-five.

9

Hormonal Pressures

Personality and Hormones

In 1983 Niels H. Lauersen, MD, and Eileen Stukane wrote a book titled *Premenstrual Syndrome and You*. These words appeared on the cover: "Over 5 million women are in the dark about a severe hormonal imbalance affecting them 10 days out of every month. They are frightened by violent fluctuations in mood, depression, and weight gain, and they don't know what's causing them."

The medical profession continues to confirm the fact that premenstrual tension definitely causes an alteration in a woman's personality. Tension begins gradually. Symptoms increase, crescendo-like, and continue progressively, accompanied by a foreboding sensation of indescribable insecurity. This is displayed by restlessness, an inability to concentrate, an unnatural and extreme annoyance with trifles, unreasonable emotional outbursts, and causeless crying spells that seem to mimic an oncoming mental disease.[1]

With all the information that has been distributed over the last few years through books, magazines, and television, I thought women could easily find answers about how monthly hormone changes affect their physical, psychological, social, and emotional life.[2] The truth is that many women aren't familiar with this information and have been told their problems are in their heads. This is poppycock! There is clear evidence that a woman's menstrual cycle can drastically affect the way she feels about herself, her husband, her children, her profession, her ministry, and so forth. You name it; it's affected.

Most women will have a monthly menstrual cycle for forty years of their lives. During each month, two ovarian hormones have great impact on a woman's emotions. Estrogen dominates the preovulation phase, and progesterone affects the postovulation phase.

Many women may have five changes in their personality within each menstrual cycle. Though the actual symptoms a woman experiences may vary from month to month, the monthly phases tend to be cyclic. I'd like to draw an analogy between these phases and the seasons of the year.

Phase 1: The Spring Phase

This phase starts with the blood flow of the menstrual cycle and is dominated by estrogen. During this time, a woman feels bright and fresh, like spring. New surges of life burst inside her. She is positive, assertive, outgoing, happy, energetic, and well coordinated. Little threatens her, and she feels she can accomplish almost anything. Her relationships with her husband and kids are delightful and relaxed. The tension she felt prior to her period vanishes, and life is a whole new ball game.

Phase 2: The Summer Phase

This is a peaceful, happy, affirming, creative time of the month. A woman has "warm fuzzies" for her family and friends and is generally pleased with life. She is a bit less assertive than in the spring phase but able to accomplish much. Her body is moving toward liberating an egg for fertilization. Estrogen continues to dominate.

Phase 3: The Midsummer Phase

Midsummer is that short time during which ovulation occurs. The egg leaves the ovary for possible fertilization. A woman usually feels euphoric, motherly, peaceful, sensual, and integrative. Everything in life seems absolutely wonderful. She loves her husband and kids, who can do no wrong. All of these feelings are influenced by progesterone production.

Phase 4: The Fall Phase

Immediately after ovulation, a woman begins to slowly lose energy as she enters the fall phase. Slight depression or the doldrums set in, and she isn't as enthusiastic about life as she was a few days ago. Suddenly her husband and children don't seem quite so lovable. Assertiveness is a thing of the past, and her confidence is droopy. It is generally suspected that during the fall and winter phases, hormone fluctuations are responsible for a host of unpleasant symptoms.

Phase 5: The Winter Phase

Winter sets in around the fourth week of the menstrual month, and many women become downright witchy. There are typical symptoms associated with this phase:

Unspiritual feelings

No concentration

Lowered reaction time

Sluggish

Needs extra sleep

Depressed, tired

Nervous tension

Irritable

Savage

Weepy

Outbursts of emotion

Jumpiness

High-strung temperament

Abnormal excitement

Manic activity

Hair-trigger temperament

Recurrent frenzy or catatonic depression

Hypermanic trends

Impaired self-control

Impaired judgment

Impaired willpower

Hazy thinking

Change in sexual behavior

Spending sprees

Striking change of behavior

Foreboding sensation of impending insecurity

Talking too much or not at all

Feeling of fatigue

Blanket-of-fog feeling

Sense of loss

Desire to be alone

Melancholia

Careless

Thoughtless

Unpunctual

Absentminded

Morbid memories

Supersensitive

Horrid

Irrational

Hateful

Shouts

Cyclic alteration of personality

Expressed resentment

Expressed hostility

Rattled

Captious

Hypercritical

Biting in speech

Lashes out for no reason

Suspicious

Jealous

Distrustful

Low self-esteem

Apprehension

Anxiety

Forgetfulness

Fretfulness

Sudden mood swings

Temper outbursts

Uptight, can't relax

Jittery and tremors

Loss of self-control

Loss of security

Frustration

Agitation

Fears of losing control

Restless energy

Lethargic

Crying over anything

Fights

No insights

Mistakes, accidents

Impulsive

Split-personality feeling

Self-depreciation

Negative attitudes to self

Negative attitudes to others

Abnormally hungry

Food binges

Salty foods desired

Tolerance for sugar

Cravings for foods

Compulsive eating

Touch-me-not attitude

Irritated whenever hungry

Fortunately, the menstrual flow is only a few days away, and a woman will feel quite different once this begins. However, some women suffer somatic symptoms like stomach cramps, backaches, or headaches after their periods start.

During the winter phase, a wife may feel very negative about her husband and say things like, "I wish I never married you in the first place. I hate my life. I might have had a great career if I had not married you." Her son might see her throw a temper tantrum simply because he left his bike in the middle of the driveway or his socks on the floor.

What are these poor males supposed to think when they face these tirades? Why is their wife and mother acting this way? Two weeks before, she was warm, charming, and making their favorite meals. Now she is crabby, feeding her face with junk food, and harping at them for every little thing they do. Who is this lady?

May I make a suggestion? Women, do yourselves a favor. Inform your husbands and older children about these five phases so they know what to expect. They are likely to think you're going crazy once a month, year after year, if they don't understand what's happening in your body. It will be much easier for them to tolerate your mood swings if they are informed.

The Slump

During my clinical practice, I noticed that women in their late thirties and early forties reported major changes in their attitudes, feelings, and health. It seemed I kept hearing the same story over and over again from scores of women. I didn't understand everything I heard, but I did believe them.

I could not imagine why energetic and very functional women were suddenly feeling lethargic and hopeless. Many were frightened about these changes and felt overwhelmed by ordinary duties they had successfully handled for years. Apparently nothing was physically wrong, but they felt they had to drag themselves through each day, just to keep going. Some wondered if they were beginning early menopause, but medical doctors said no, then handed the women antidepressants and told them to see a counselor or psychiatrist.

Now we understand more about the emotional phases of a woman's life. Typical symptoms associated with hormonal changes during the late thirties and early forties are:

• Drop in energy level that seems a nuisance

- A dragging feeling on some days
- A listless feeling on some days
- Loss of interest or need for sex—some say it's boring
- Earlier interests don't seem important anymore
- Boredom with duties
- Mild depression unrelated to menstrual cycle
- The blahs
- Foreboding feelings on some days
- Morbid or sad feelings on some days
- Overreaction to small irritations
- Touchiness
- Weepiness
- Feelings of craziness ("I'm bursting apart at the seams!")
- Difficulty in making small or large decisions
- Memory lapses
- Feelings of failure
- Feeling unneeded or useless
- Spiritual worries ("I wonder if I'm really a Christian.")
- Fantasies about a true love yet to emerge
- Interest in romantic novels and love stories
- Compulsive buying
- Increase of daydreaming—fantasies of escape from the present
- Recapitulation feelings ("If only I could live my life over again.")
- Regrets over past decisions or choices
- Worry over past mistakes
- Increased introspection
- Concerns about early menopause

Not long ago, I took this list of symptoms and surveyed over seventy-five women in the Northwest. The five symptoms that most frequently bothered these women were: (1) a sudden drop in energy, (2) unusual irritability, (3) touchiness/overreacting, (4) mild depression, and (5) loss of interest in highly valued activities.

It Wasn't in Her Head

Many years ago a forty-one-year-old husband sought counsel from me concerning his wife's health. He had six lovely children and told me his wife was a wonderful person. Yet he was worried.

"I work two jobs in order to feed eight of us. We both agree Margaret shouldn't work while the children are growing up. Even though my hours are long, I'm basically content with my lot in life. Margaret seemed to feel the same way, until recently."

"Do you mean she had a sudden change of attitude?" I inquired.

"That's hard to answer," he replied. "I feel like saying yes *and* no to your question."

I probed further. "Can you remember an event or crisis that preceded her changes?"

"I guess I first noticed she was acting different last summer at a family reunion. This is a great affair that Margaret looks forward to every year. It's the only time all her family is together in one large group.

"Last summer she seemed happy about the upcoming reunion and cooked three days straight to prepare for the event. But, Mrs. Lush, the strangest thing happened at that party. When we were all together at lunch, she suddenly flew into a rage over something she was discussing with her favorite sister. Her tirade went on and on. I was stunned, because I had never seen her act that way. The incident ruined the party for Margaret, and she felt totally humiliated by her overreaction. She and her sister later talked and worked things out between themselves.

"That was nearly a year ago. Since then she has seemed rather listless, with little energy or interest in things around her. She cries a lot and says nobody needs her. But, Mrs. Lush, that isn't true. She's the center of our family, and we all love her very much.

"Margaret used to be a garage-sale and flea-market buff. She made beautiful crafts and enjoyed being creative in the kitchen. Now, she doesn't seem to care about doing anything. Please, Mrs. Lush, tell me how I can help her."

I have never forgotten this honest plea for help. A week later I met with Margaret, and her story duplicated her husband's. I wondered if the picnic incident was causing her present low spirits, but concluded that it wasn't that simple. There was more to the picture than I could see. I was stumped. Something was happening that I didn't understand.

After this case, I watched and listened to women in their late thirties and early forties in a new way. After many years of clinical investigation, I started to broadcast my findings with Dr. James Dobson. His radio program, "Focus on the Family," was flooded with responses from the listening audience, and the phone calls and letters continue to come.

One woman called from the East Coast after hearing the broadcast. Extremely upset, she said, "I have just heard your broadcast, and your descriptions fit me. There are times when life seems unbearable. I feel like I have crazy days. Some mornings I wake up and feel like I'm losing my mind!"

When she said she was forty-three, I thought, *That figures.*
I told her I had heard this from numerous other women in
their early forties, and I tried to offer encouragement.

"I know what you are experiencing, and you are not going
crazy. Your body is going through some changes and influ-
encing your mind to make you think you are going crazy. I
know the scary feelings you have are very real, and not loony
fantasies. These panic attacks may be closely associated with
hormonal fluctuations that occur in women during their late
thirties and early forties."

"Oh!" she exclaimed. "You mean my body is sending these
crazy ideas to my mind, and my mind isn't really crazy after
all?"

"Yes, that's right," I replied.

"Well, that's the best news I've heard in months. I can
live with that much easier than thinking I'm going out of
my mind!"

I assured her that if that were the case, hundreds of other
women who called me were going crazy, too. For further
information, see my book, *Emotional Phases of a Woman's
Life.* This book explores the various phases of a woman's
life, examining the hormonal changes that at times seem
to govern her body and mind. As each phase is discussed,
hope and help is offered to those who feel victimized by
their hormones.

Postpartum Challenges

The coming of a new baby has been announced. This is no
ordinary baby; it is my first great-grandchild. I told my granddaughter, "I hope you have twins, but if you don't, you must
have another baby right away, because this baby belongs to
the whole clan. You know what they say to royal mothers:

The first is the heir . . . the second is the spare . . . the third is yours." My son, who will be the baby's grand-uncle, said, "Mother this is an international event for our family. After the death of our beloved Poppa, we all need this baby."

This baby, barely a few months into its development, has stirred all kinds of excitement. My granddaughter and her husband are ecstatic, and everyone in the family is saying, "We can't stand the suspense." All vacation plans scheduled during the month of the baby's arrival have been canceled. The baby's father, a physician, has planned a short leave of absence from the hospital. I was told, "Nana, make sure you don't have any conferences scheduled the month I'm due to deliver."

Obviously this baby is going to be showered with love and affection, and my granddaughter will have more support than the average new mother, but will she escape the typical blues that follow childbirth? No. Not even her joy or the support of her welcoming family can rule out the possibility of mood swings. Why? Because she is female and her hormones will sometimes rule the roost.

Those who have researched postpartum mood disorders tell us that up to 80 percent of women may experience mood changes after giving birth. These can range from mild feelings of sadness and irritability to incapacitating symptoms of depression and psychosis.[3] Medical experts identify four different levels of mood disturbance. Postpartum blues affect at least one-half of birthing women. Most people refer to them as the "baby blues." They set in within a week after birth and usually last a few days. The cause of this depression is not fully understood, but some endocrinologists suggest it is related to the profound drop in progesterone levels immediately after birth. Breast-feeding can be helpful because prolactin, the mothering hormone released during breast-feeding, seems to have a calming effect on the mother.

The baby blues must be distinguished from a more serious condition called postpartum depression, which may last a year or more. Approximately 10 to 20 percent of mothers experience this disorder in the first three months after childbirth. Postpartum depression is characterized by disruption of appetite, insomnia, and inability to concentrate, suicidal thoughts, and a plunge in self-esteem. This depression can occur suddenly, without warning, or it can be associated with other life stresses. However, in some cases there is no apparent outside cause for the depression. Occasionally doctors will prescribe antidepressants or minor tranquilizers to help the mother cope. Usually the symptoms subside in a few months, whether or not medication is prescribed.[4]

Postpartum anxiety disorder is characterized by long periods of feeling anxious, tense, and jittery. Other symptoms include difficulty falling asleep, sweating, blushing, dizziness, palpitations, muscle tension, and a foreboding sense of worry. In a postpartum psychosis, a mother loses touch with reality. This rarely occurs.

Reports about severe postpartum disturbances are more common in recent years than when I first began counseling. I cannot help wondering if young mothers are pressured by our culture to feel they must snap back to a normal routine, including hard work, much too soon.

When I was growing up, it was the custom to either go home to mother or to a relative for a time of recuperation. We were never expected to immediately resume our normal activities. We were pampered, spoiled, and allowed to feel special.

I don't see this happening much now. Young mothers boast about how fast they return to work. I hear, "I had my baby on Friday and was in church the following Sunday morning," or, "I was back to work three weeks after delivery." I don't understand why some think this is important. The baby has hardly had time to settle down and learn to breast-feed.

The birth of a child is much more than a simple biological event. It ushers in a new developmental phase in a woman's life. I had the feeling I was making history with the birth of each new child. I think it is absolutely natural to experience a letdown after we have been high for months, anticipating the birth of the baby.

Dr. Julia Sherman suggests we can minimize postpartum reactions by planning ahead for sufficient help and rest. Dr. Michael O'Hara and Dr. Jane Engeldinger offer ten suggestions that can help forestall emotional distress after delivery.[5]

- Reassure yourself that postpartum blues are normal, and may reflect the effects of exhaustion and relief of built-up tension from delivery, or the initial adjustment to coping with the demands of a newborn.
- Having a baby is a shared responsibility. Women whose spouses are supportive and physically helpful are less likely to become depressed after delivery.
- Seek help and advice from women more experienced in child care to reduce excessive or unnecessary worrying over routine matters. Find a confidante with whom you can share your concerns and worries. Confide in your partner, too.
- Learn to say "NO!" and protect your time. The time necessary to care for a newborn is always greater than expected.
- Whenever possible, avoid major life changes such as moving, changing jobs, or assuming care of relatives.

- Get plenty of rest. Sleep deprivation can have a dev-
  astating effect on mood and coping ability. Spouses
  should care for the infant when possible to allow the
  mother to rest.

- Learn to adjust your standards for activities (e.g., time
  with spouse and other children, neatness of the house,
  time on the job). Trying to maintain the same level of
  performance in all activities in addition to caring for
  a newborn can lead to exhaustion and frustration.

- Avoid isolation after the baby is born. Make arrangements for personal time to exercise, shop, visit with
  friends, or just relax.

- Arrange for a pediatrician before delivery so that medical advice is readily available.

- Know whom you can contact if you are having emotional problems after delivery. Make contact when
  necessary. Usually your obstetrician and/or family
  physician should be available for consultation. Other
  resources might include a counselor, local postpartum
  support groups, or mental health professionals.

My daughter, Heather, received midwifery training in New
Zealand after completing her BS degree in nursing. Even
with all her knowledge about babies and physiology, I clearly
remember her emergency phone call to my office when her
baby was about seven days old. She yelled, "Mother, get over
here to my house *now!*" I darted out of the counseling office, leaving all my appointments to be canceled. I couldn't
imagine what had caused her hysteria. When I arrived at
her home, she screamed through her tears, "Mother, you
can *have* this baby!" She had bottomed out in depression
and simply could not cope. She needed me, and you can be
sure I stayed with her until the phase passed. A few days

later she was back to her old self again. These types of experiences after giving birth are reported by women around the world. They are also mentioned by women who have had their tubes tied.

The Impact of Tubal Ligation

Tubal sterilization is one of the most frequently performed surgical operations. For women whose families are complete, it is the most popular method of contraception. Increasing numbers of younger women are now requesting the surgery.[6]

Some women feel pressured into the surgery. They consent to the operation even though they would rather not. I've known of many cases where husbands pushed their wives to have their tubes tied because they didn't want the responsibility of birth control or the financial burdens of additional children. Sometimes their marriage was in trouble and one or both felt insecure about the future. Under the pressure of the moment, cutting the tubes seemed like a good thing to do. However, if a divorce and remarriage followed, the wives were unable to have children with their new spouses. This led to intense feelings of guilt and regret. I've known many women who mourned for years after robbing themselves of the chance to have more children. Some can't accept their loss because their ability to reproduce was the most important part of their female identity.[7]

There are those who complain of abrupt changes in their menstrual cycle following tubal sterilization. They say their doctors don't take them seriously, and they are told there is a lack of research in this area.

Even the medical community confirms the possible adverse effects of tubal sterilization on menstruation. The incidence of menstrual disturbance following tubal ligations has been reported to vary from 25 percent to 60 percent.[8]

I suggest that much tension is generated from the physiological changes that follow this surgery. Women should not be lightly dismissed when they report complaints. I also advise women to counsel with an expert before finalizing their decision about sterilization.

I recall one young mother with six children. Her doctor advised permanent sterilization because she conceived easily, even while using birth control. Knowing the family was under great financial strain, he didn't bill the woman for his services. She was deeply grateful for the procedure and relieved that she couldn't bear any more children. However, she was depressed for several months after the surgery.

There may be a physical explanation for this. Medical research is inconclusive about this issue, but there are some experts who are willing to speculate. Dr. Penny Wise Budoff says a tubal ligation may interfere with the blood supply to the ovaries and lead to abnormal hormone production. A blood-deprived ovary may no longer function perfectly, or its hormonal output may be decreased, making ovulation irregular.[9] Dr. Katharina Dalton suggests that less progesterone is produced by the ovaries following the surgery.[10]

Some physicians say it has not been scientifically proven that tubal ligations are linked to depression. Numerous women have told me their doctors said their depression was "all in their head," or due to regrets about having the surgery. I cannot settle for these simple answers. I can't help but think there is a biological connection. We do know that postpartum changes and sterilization do seem to put women under unusual stress and tension, however.

10

Menopause

Menopause is a time of highs, lows, and other annoying symptoms that can leave us feeling baffled, angry, tense, and depressed.

When I was young, I heard gruesome stories from other girls about the dreaded "change of life." Such things bothered me, so I asked Mother if the stories were true.

"Whoever told you such silly stories?" she responded. "You are far too young to have ideas like that in your head. I never heard such things until after I was married."

For some reason grown-ups in my day left many things unsaid, creating mystery in my mind about selected subjects. I learned quickly not to ask certain questions, if I didn't want to be reprimanded.

It is interesting how differently society views menopause now, compared to the first half of the century. Helene Deutsch, a famous psychoanalyst in the early 1900s, wrote two volumes on the psychology of women. She painted a dismal picture of midlife: "When the expulsion of the ova from the ovary ceases, woman has ended her existence as bearer of a new future and has reached her natural end; her partial death as servant of the species stops. She now struggles against decline. She feels the fatal touch of death itself."[1]

Deutsch viewed menopause as a time of declining functions, disappointment, and mortification. After menopause, she said, "a woman's activity thrust outside the home is only a protest and compensation against the decline she feels within."[2]

Years later we hear a vastly different perspective from Therese Benedek, who published one of the world's greatest books on the psychosexual functions of women. She views menopause as a great developmental phase that ushers a woman into her peak time of life. Benedek says:

> Internal physiological changes will stimulate psychological processes which will now enable women to master new things. 85% of all women pass through menopause without interruption of their daily routine. Once free from the reproductive cycle, the body has new energies to devote to new tasks. This results in a more balanced personality which finds new aims for its psychic energy, and releases new impetus for learning. [3]

Benedek isn't alone in her observations. Others in the field are proposing that women experience a kind of rebirth after menopause, too.[4] I have found this to be true in my life; however, getting through menopause and on to the rebirth was no easy task.

The Only Way Is Through It

When I was a young teenager, my parents took a long sea voyage to America. Father was going to be awarded the

Carnegie Trust Fellowship from America and an opportunity to study American methods of agricultural education. My mother's health had been poor, and Father wanted her to accompany him for six months of the trip.

During the long sea voyage, my mother never had a regular menstrual period. This caused some alarm, and as soon as they landed, she visited an American doctor who informed her that she had suddenly passed through menopause. She was in excellent health. Mother had a wonderful time in the United States and came home a changed person. After menopause she never suffered with the asthma attacks that had plagued her for years.

All the horror stories I had logged during my childhood were put to rest when I heard of Mother's experience. I expected to go through menopause much the same. Unfortunately, things didn't turn out that way.

Mother went through menopause in her early forties. I went through it in my early fifties, and believe me, I was weird. I was extremely depressed, worried obsessively about my children, and lacked all reasonable judgment about their lives. I interfered too much and was a total nuisance.

My son, David, a new medical doctor, finally dragged me to an experienced family doctor for an exam. He discovered that my estrogen level was almost nonexistent and treated the depletion. I was astounded by the miraculous changes that occurred. I continued the treatment for a year, and the deep depression, warped judgment, and obsessive thinking never returned.

For most women, the journey through menopause is not smooth. It reminds me of one of my flights to the East Coast. I often fly over the Rocky Mountains to speak at conferences in the eastern United States. One trip was extremely rough. As the plane swooshed up and down, my face turned pale and my anxieties surged. I had been on bumpy flights before, but these weren't your average bumps. It felt as if the plane were rocketing toward the moon one minute and plunging out of control toward earth the next. I couldn't contain my fears and called for an attendant.

The hostess reassured me there was nothing wrong with the plane. "Rough travel is always expected in this particular area because of the mountains. We are experiencing down drafts, but there is no danger whatsoever. It won't be long before the turbulence ends and we'll have a smooth flight again."

Her words brought peace. The turbulence was expected, we weren't out of control, and there was no danger. Such is the trip through menopause.

Thousands of women need basic information about the connection between their minds and bodies. Let's look at the facts.

During a woman's childbearing years, the production of ovarian hormones remains at a high peak. Toward middle life, the ovaries become less active as their production of hormones falls off, and conception becomes less likely. Menstrual cycles become less marked and more irregular. Finally menstruation ceases altogether. This gradual departure of ovarian hormones is known as menopause.[5]

The reproductive years are approximately ages thirteen to fifty-three. We now know that there are slow changes or hormonal shifts that begin in the mid-thirties, when the hormonal output is at a peak. One well-known expert on this subject, Dr. Penny Wise Budoff, says, "There is a transitional phase when ovarian function and its hormonal production are declining. The decline of ovarian function goes on for years."[6]

The Phases of Menopause

I am often asked the question, "Do you think menopause occurs in stages?" My answer is a strong perhaps, but I must allow for the fact that women are all very different.

During the long transition and slow decline of hormonal production, there is one marked period between the ages of thirty-eight and forty-three when women experience definite changes. I refer to this as the malaise phase, which is the early beginning of the countdown toward the final close of the reproductive years.

Following this phase, many women, but not all, report improvements and say they feel better. Then comes a phase doctors refer to as early menopause. Symptoms in this phase may appear any time during the forties, and they vary from one woman to the next. These are the symptoms usually reported during early menopause:

Irregular menstrual periods

Varying intervals between periods

Flow increase or decrease

Occasional flooding

An upset endocrine system

Variation in cycle length

Marked wide mood swings

Severe PMS symptoms

Hot flashes

Poor judgment

Obsession with certain people

Fatigue

Headaches

Irritability

Emotional attachment to physician

Unexplained depression

After a woman passes through the midlife malaise and early phase of menopause, she is ushered into the time of life when her reproductive system completely shuts down. This is what doctors refer to as menopause. Fluctuating emotions are the norm during this phase and may continue beyond the time menstruation stops. Following are some of the symptoms of menopause.

Emotional Symptoms of Menopause

- Unaccountable mood swings
- Fear of losing attractiveness
- Binge eating
- Lack of emotional security
- Preoccupation with body
- Frustration
- Crawling-skin sensation
- Fear of aging
- Diminished capacity to love
- Loss of sense of wholeness
- Tension from family worries
- Perfectionism
- Obsession with kids' problems
- Fluctuating sense of well-being
- Loss of objectivity
- Poor judgment
- Low self-esteem
- Sense of futility
- Aggressiveness and hostility
- Mental imbalance
- Headaches
- Tenseness
- Narrowing interests
- Fear of the unknown
- Dependency
- Reappearance of old resentments
- Inappropriate responses
- Depression
- Negative attitudes
- Irritability
- Nervousness
- Melancholia
- Feelings of suffocation
- Unpleasant reactions
- Restlessness
- Loss of energy

Feelings of sadness or loss
Withdrawal
Dissatisfaction
Easily offended
Looks for slights
Desire for peace and quiet or rest
Self-accusation
Crying jags
Trivial worries seem big
Regressive behavior
Egotism
Narcissism
Frigidity (for some)
Lack of concentration

Somatic Symptoms of Menopause

Excessive fatigue
Breathlessness
Giddiness
Dizziness
Constipation
Diarrhea
Breast pain
Heavy flow
Hot flashes
Insomnia
Decreased energy
Atrophy of breasts and genital tissue
Uterus and vagina become smaller
Thinner vaginal mucus, more infections
Tingling extremities
Painful intercourse
Loss of hair
Muscle weakness and stiffening
Bone loss due to osteoporosis
Atrophic arthritis
Build-up of cholesterol
Hypertension
Estrogen loss disrupts whole system
Diabetes
Disruption of digestive and vascular systems
Headaches
Crawling-skin sensation
Night sweats
Heart palpitations
Weight gain
Severe premenstrual tension
Eating binges

Some Facts on Menopause[7]

In our country today we have over 40 million women who have safely made the transition from premenopause to postmenopause. You might be interested in some statistics I've gathered on menopause.

The average age of cessation of menstrual function is 52 years. About 30 percent of women will have had menopause by the time they are 45, and 98 percent will have had menopause by the time they are 55.[8]

It is estimated that 75 to 80 percent of women will develop symptoms caused by estrogen withdrawal.

Premenopause can begin as early as 35 or be delayed until the age of 60. The average range is between 45 and 55. Women whose menses stop before 45 years of age are said to have a premature menopause.

Individuals vary greatly in when premenopause begins and the length of time it takes for the transition to be complete. There are some factors, though, that may indicate whether you will have an early or late menopause.

Some sources say there is no connection between when a woman starts her menses and when menses end. Yet Katharina Dalton, in her book *Once a Month*, says there is. She says those who start menstruation early tend to finish late, and those who begin late tend to finish early.[9]

Women who have had a lifetime of low estrogen output, Dr. Dalton says, "have a tendency to finish menstruation before the average. On the other hand PMS sufferers usually finish after 50 years of age."[10]

There may be some genetic factors involved, too. A family of women—mother, daughter, sister, aunt—may all end their menstrual cycles early or late. This is unusual, however, and I've found you can't really count on similarity among family members.

According to Dr. Dalton, a survey of forty-eight- to forty-nine-year-old postmenopausal women found that a high percentage were smokers. This suggests that smoking could lead to earlier menopause.[11]

Basically, the effect of estrogen loss depends largely on your own genetic resistance to aging, your overall health, quality of diet, and activity.

Physical Symptoms of Menopause

Now it's time to have a closer look at some of the somatic (physical) symptoms associated with menopause.

Erratic Menstrual Cycles

A woman might experience a very gradual ending, where periods are regular but last for fewer days. Another woman may complain of erratic periods, missing one occasionally and then gradually missing more and more. For some women, like my mother, there may be a sudden cessation of menstruation.

Hot Flashes or Flushes

These are burning sensations usually beginning from the waist and moving to the top of the head. Outwardly the skin might be flushed and beads of sweat may appear. Along with the flush, a woman might have a fluttering in the chest or palpitations, apprehension, or anxiety attacks. A flush will last only a few minutes. They may range from one to two a week up to one hundred a day. This is one of the most common complaints of premenopausal women and is often the source of much embarrassment.

129

Hot flashes frequently occur at night. The flush is uncomfortable, and the woman awakens to find herself completely drenched. This phenomenon is referred to as night sweats.

Insomnia and Consequent Tiredness

This is a common complaint as well, and may be due to sleepless nights resulting from hot flashes or other premenopausal problems, as well as emotional upsets.

Vaginal Dryness

Dryness and atrophy of the genital tissue may be due to a lack of estrogen. This may lead to vaginitis, itching, irritation of the vaginal area, pain, urinary frequency, and pain during intercourse. These symptoms may cause a decreased interest in sex.

Bladder Changes

The bladder and bladder opening become thinner. The bladder may not empty properly. This condition can lead to cystitis (urinary tract infections) and leaking. The muscle that holds urine in often becomes weak, and a simple cough or sneeze releases an unexpected flood of urine.

Loss of Fatty Tissue and Decreased Muscle Tone

This may lead to a collapse of vaginal walls. Occasionally women end up with a prolapsed uterus, which may require reparative surgery.

Dry Skin

The skin often becomes dry, pale, and thin, losing its elasticity, which contributes to wrinkling, especially around the eyes, mouth, and neck.

Breast Changes

Breasts may sag from a decrease in fat cells and muscle tone.

Unusual Skin Sensations

One rather odd symptom that's been reported by premenopausal women is a creepy-crawly sensation on the skin. In a letter I received recently, a pastor's wife shared a story about a friend whose cat is being treated for a hormone deficiency because she was spayed too young. "The cat kept pulling her fur out with her teeth, thinking that things were crawling on her skin," she writes. "The cat has to take hormones! Maybe I ought to go to a veterinarian for my scalp condition!" Sad to think that felines at times get more attention and better treatment than women.

Other Symptoms

Often related to estrogen deficiency are dizziness, weight gain, bloating, and gastrointestinal disturbances such as constipation and diarrhea.

Calcium Deficiency

Low or fluctuating calcium levels may bring on osteoporosis, and arthritic-like pains may develop in the bones. Women in premenopause often complain of joint stiffness and leg cramps. These pains may be due to a lack of calcium.

More on Osteoporosis

Estrogen deficiency has been linked to a progressive and serious bone disease called osteoporosis. Lately there has been much literature written on osteoporosis. Today it is a widely accepted theory that much of the bone deterioration seen in postmenopausal women in their seventies is due to a lack of estrogen.

Researchers now feel that problems such as shortened, deformed, and misaligned spines; the "dowager's hump," or bow at the top of the spine; and fragile bones that lead to frequent fractures can often be lessened with estrogen replacement therapy.

Symptoms Vary

Again, not everyone goes through premenopause in the same way. Dr. Penny Wise Budoff, in her book *No More Menstrual Cramps and Other Good News*, says:

> There is a marked individual variation in the amount and proportion of the remaining hormones the ovaries produce, as well as in the total length of time that this occurs. This is why some women have severe symptoms, while others have few complaints.
>
> Women with more fat tend to be able to convert more androstenedione to estrogen and have fewer symptoms. Some women may never become symptomatic: they may produce hormones over a longer period of time and have a slower waning of the entire process.[12]

Let's take a look at the emotional upheaval often accompanying the fluctuating hormone levels in premenopausal women.

Growing Older: Growing Better

Unfortunately, premenopause directly coincides with or follows midlife malaise. Let's face it: menopause couldn't happen at a more inconvenient time. Unfortunately, in many women the feelings about menopause are not happy ones. Perhaps they haven't yet been able to let go of the dream of youth. Perhaps they haven't yet come to the other side of midlife. Whatever the cause, they come into premenopause uncertain, unsure of their roles, and frightened about the future.

Paula, a woman of fifty-five, married for twenty-five years with four children, decided one day to run away from home with a man fifteen years younger than herself. "She had been growing increasingly restless," her husband told me. "I should have seen trouble coming when she started dressing differently. She wore more makeup, dressed more like a girl in her teens than a woman. Then one day she just announced she was leaving. She said I was too old for her, that this guy made her feel young again."

Paula was trying to fight for her youth. One day she'll wake up to find that age has won the battle after all. I've never been able to understand this obsession to hold on to youth.

Actually, society has recently been entertaining the notion that older people can be beautiful. There has been a lot of attention given to glamorous women over forty—women like Linda Evans, Jane Fonda, Joan Collins, and *The Golden Girls* of the weekly television program. In a way, this is great. We see role models and positive affirmations of older people achieving and maintaining success.

The new vision of what a woman over forty can be creates a few problems, though. These older television women flaunt their good looks, sex appeal, and the fact that they are over forty and still gorgeous. These women, as portrayed for all the world to see, are rich and beautiful, adored by men of all ages, have no hot flashes, depression, snappy moods, or crying spells and appear wonderfully in control of their lives and their men.

Nevertheless, as on TV, there are many women who have successfully transitioned through their mid-life malaise. They are revived, reborn, and ready to move on with fresh goals. They actually look forward to growing older and seem perfectly happy as they watch their hair gray and their wrinkles deepen. There is a sparkle in their eyes as their children's offspring call them Grandma.

Yet for each woman who ages happily and gracefully, there are half a dozen who mourn every birthday past forty. They bring out the black balloons, black T-shirts, black coffee cups, all covered with sayings like "I'm over the hill."

I hate that saying. For one thing, I don't believe a word of it. Life doesn't stop at forty—it *starts*. That's when climbing the mountain of life really gets interesting!

The Emotional Side of Menopause

Emotional stresses arise when women don't understand the association between their strange emotional upsets and their hormonal imbalance. Although emotions can and often are separate from our hormones, they can also be very much connected.

Emotions fluctuate, as do the changing hormone levels. They vary from woman to woman, depending on mental and physical health, attitudes, background, and relationships.

Even those who suffer the full course of symptoms generally survive. Menopause, after all, is not fatal; but it certainly can be frustrating.

Often women suffer needlessly, when with understanding, proper treatment, and a physician's care, they could lead a normal life. It is important for us to go into menopause with a feeling of self-worth, knowing our lives are not ending as we pass through this transition, but that a new and exciting phase is beginning.

The emotional and hormonal instability during menopause is the bad news. The good news is: eventually, it will end. The even better news is that with estrogen therapy, the premenopausal and postmenopausal years don't have to play havoc with our lives.

Menopause is nothing to be afraid of. I sort of looked forward to it, and I hope you will, too. It's simply one of those rocks in life that we must either climb over or find a way around. Since there is no way around menopause, I suggest you take a deep breath and commence climbing.

The Aftermath of Hysterectomy

During the later years of my work as a marriage and family therapist, I saw a tremendous number of marriages dissolve when couples were in their forties. The case histories showed that a high percentage of the women in these marriages had a hysterectomy within two years prior to the divorce. I had heard all the standard explanations given by therapists for these marital breakdowns, but I wasn't satisfied. I wondered if something more was going on that wasn't being identified. Could there have been some kind of delayed depression that surfaced a year or so after their surgeries, something biochemical in nature?

Many women report delayed depression following a hysterectomy. When their surgeons say they are recovering nicely and that they need to develop a more positive attitude, these women feel like guilty failures. Scores of women have told me their doctors thought their symptoms were all in their head.

Two recent surveys have documented a high incidence of depression among women after a hysterectomy. In many cases this depression occurs about three years after the hysterectomy, whether or not the ovaries were removed.[13] When delivering a paper at the Royal Society of Medicine in London, Dr. Katharina Dalton said, "44% of the women studied had been divorced, separated, or had sought the assistance of a Marriage Counselor since their hysterectomy." She identified two types of posthysterectomy depression: cyclical depression and continuous depression. Cyclical depression comes and goes, with periods of relief. Continuous depression remains, without intermittent periods of relief. Dr. Donald Richards, a general medical practitioner in Oxford, England, also found a high incidence of depression among those surveyed after a hysterectomy.[14]

Managing Menopause[15]

Years ago, women suffering with premenopausal symptoms were simply ignored unless their symptoms became serious enough for them to be sent to a psychiatrist, where they would often be given tranquilizers or at times even shock therapy.

Today, at least among the more up-to-date family practitioners and gynecologists, menopause is considered a "disease process" that must be followed up by medical care in order to prevent a series of life-threatening maladies such as osteoporosis. I thoroughly dislike using the word *disease* in connection with menopause. I'd rather think of it as a developmental phase. Still, I suppose we shouldn't worry too much about what the medical profession calls it, as long as they do something about it.

Most doctors see medical intervention as a must, unless their patient is producing adequate amounts of estrogen on her own. In this section we'll examine the various treatments and helps for women in the premenopausal phase of their lives.

See Your Doctor

If you suspect you are entering menopause—especially if you are having a difficult time with some of the symptoms we discussed—I'd recommend an examination.

Learn all you can about menopause and the appropriate and generally accepted forms of treatment before you go. Then feel free to discuss your symptoms. Find out what your doctor's approach is to menopause. How does he feel about it? What is his attitude? How does he treat his menopausal patients?

In order to evaluate your doctor, ask him to explain menopause to you. You'll be able to tell if he really cares for you and will work with you or if he considers premenopausal women a pain in his cervical vertebrae.

If you feel uncomfortable with the doctor, if he doesn't give you adequate explanations, if he doesn't believe in estrogen therapy, or if he takes you and your problems too lightly, get a second opinion.

Diet, Exercise, and Other Necessary Helps

If you have not already reviewed your eating habits and exercise program, I suggest you do so now. Naturally, the way we take care of our bodies in the first half of our lives will directly affect how our bodies treat us during the second half. Unfortunately, we have to live with the logical consequences of our actions.

It's not too late, however. Shaping up your body and your eating habits can make your mature years happier, healthier, and more fun.

Exercise is especially important to us as we grow older. It improves circulation and, according to one of my sources, "Next to estrogen and calcium, weight-bearing exercise [walking, jogging, bicycling, jumping rope] appears to be the most important technique for preserving bone. Exercise actually stimulates the formation of new bone in a woman's body."[16]

One special exercise I encourage you to do on a regular basis is Kegel exercises. This exercise tightens up the muscles in the vaginal area. Relaxed, loose, or damaged muscle tissue can result in a prolapsed uterus. Kegels not only help to prevent this problem, but also works to minimize urine leakage.

To do Kegels, simply tighten up the muscle (as you would to stop the flow of urine) and hold it for about two seconds. It may help to think in terms of tightening or pulling in and holding the whole bottom.

Sound simple? There's a catch: Kegels only work with repetition—about three hundred times a day. No one knows you're doing them, however, so you can pull in that bottom any place, any time. You may want to try doing it in groups of twenty-five to fifty at a time.

Help for Vaginal Dryness

Lack of estrogen can cause a drying out of vaginal tissues and skin. Feel free to use lotions and lubricants on skin surfaces as needed. Also, you may want to keep some Vaseline or K-Y Jelly handy to prevent painful intercourse.

Vaginal dryness may not be relieved entirely by estrogen tablets. If not, an estrogen cream is available for local application. You may want to ask your doctor about it if painful intercourse, vaginal dryness, and itching are a problem for you.

Don't We Live in a Wonderful World?

We no longer have to put up with unexplained tension and stress, hot flashes, painful intercourse, or any of the other symptoms that make life miserable for the menopausal woman. Not that all our troubles are over, but at least they are made easier to bear. We can have better health, both mentally and physically, as we move into the best phase of all: postmenopause.

PART TWO

TYPICAL
RESPONSES
TO TENSION

11

The Role of Early Conditioning

I bet he felt foolish, walking around the backyard with baby ducks following him. He flapped his arms like wings, and they imitated him. What would the neighbors have said, had they seen him? Yet it won him a Nobel Prize in 1973.

Konrad Lorenz was a zoologist studying animal behavior. He raised baby ducks as part of his experimentation. Just as the eggs began to hatch, he quickly removed Mama Duck and placed himself next to the ducklings, who bonded to him as though he were Mom. When he waddled across the yard, they followed. They tried to go everywhere he went. However, as the ducklings matured, a noticeable problem set them apart: they did not waddle normally. Because Lorenz was unable to exactly imitate a duck's waddle, his progeny never learned the correct procedure. They were indeed odd ducks, because they had bonded to a man and patterned their behavior on him instead of on their natural mother.

This led to the discovery that ducks and other animals have developmental timetables for learning and refining certain behaviors that are common to their species. Ducks have a developmental timetable of only a few hours after birth in which to bond to their mother and learn to be proper ducks. Not having a mother duck available, Lorenz's ducks bonded to him and never developed properly. It was also learned that the developed behavior could not be established before or after a certain range of time. If Lorenz placed the mother by her ducklings hours after birth, the ducklings developed normally, but replacement had to occur during a particular developmental time.

The process of fully establishing behavioral patterns or traits became known as imprinting. The ducks imprinted on Lorenz instead of Mom. The imprint, or brand of his influence, was firmly established during that critical time.[1]

Lorenz's findings are helpful in explaining our own early conditioning. We handle tension in ways that we learned while growing up in our families. My bent toward avoiding negative emotions and conflict didn't happen by accident; I was conditioned to respond this way.

In my youth, ladies were to speak with a well-modulated, controlled, pleasant voice. They were never to gabble, speak fast, or run their words together, displaying excitement or anxiety. Under no circumstances were they to show negative feelings.

Men were permitted to show anger; it was a sign of masculinity. However, true aristocrats didn't reveal their feelings, considering it best to keep others guessing about what was going on in their minds. I learned many of these lessons from home and some from a marvelous story about Lady Brownley that I read in our third-grade *Weekly Reader*. Seventy years later, I remember the story as if I had read it yesterday.

Lord and Lady Brownley lived in a castle with a large staff that tended the farm and beautiful gardens. Lord and Lady Brownley's only son was destined to inherit the estate and a seat in the House of Lords.

During World War I, England was unprepared for war; hordes of untrained soldiers were sent to the trenches in France. Young Brownley enlisted with the men on the estate, and Lady Brownley offered her services as a Red Cross nurse, caring for wounded soldiers in a London hospital. The casualties came in by the hundreds each day, and Lady Brownley worked long hours with the other nurses, allowing herself no special privileges because of her rank.

One morning when she was on duty in the emergency dormitory, a uniformed messenger walked into the hospital waving a telegram. He said, "I am told Lady Brownley is here. I must give her this message." Everyone stopped and stared at the black-banded telegram. Lady Brownley tore open the envelope to find that her son had been killed. She swayed and was about to lose her balance when two nurses rushed to her aid. They told her they would send for a Red Cross car to take her home immediately. Her reply became a famous saying I will never forget: "No. I will not turn aside from my duty. I will complete my shift. The living must serve the living."

Her strong stoicism still affects me today. Actually, I am not a true stoic, because I don't sternly repress all emotion or condemn personal pleasure. A pure stoic never complains and is indifferent to pleasure and pain. I see myself more as being brave, unwilling to whine, and somewhat guarded with my feelings.

I learned my lessons well during my early life. The day of my first menstrual period, Mother took me aside to explain what was happening and then said sternly, "You are never to discuss this with your friends. Only low-class girls talk about menstruation." I concluded that conversations about my body were completely off-limits, especially in mixed company.

My Grandmother Hilton thought her sisters were inferior and weak in character because they talked about their illnesses. My father had the highest admiration for Grandmother Hilton. I made special note of what he esteemed.

Mother, Father, and Grandmother Hilton were power people in my life. I gave them power, and they influenced me. Throughout life there are certain people whom we adore or admire. Perhaps they are heroes we read about or see on the screen. Perhaps they are historic figures or characters found in books. They may even be our own family members. Those we esteem make an impression on us.

While power people may bring out the best in us, they may also cause stress in our lives. We may strive so hard to be what we think they want us to be that we lose sight of our own personal desires and goals. This can lead to feelings of inferiority that last a lifetime. I always felt inferior to my mother, but at the same time her high standards positively influenced my life.

My early years were wonderful. Life was safe, secure, and good in every way. Mother and Father were remarkable people with a long heritage of stable families. I was surrounded by outstanding role models. As a result, my early conditioning was more powerful and fixed than some. I accepted everything around me as right and excellent. I had no reason to challenge my training. In my mind, my superiors were superior. I strove to be self-controlled and stoic. I remember putting myself through endurance tests to challenge my inner strength. I didn't let others know me; I kept all my feelings to myself. If I felt sick, I did my best to overcome the illness without others knowing it. Complaining wasn't acceptable.

Any negative feelings were to be invisible. Anger was simply not permitted. I suppressed it. To this day I have to guard myself against this tendency.

In time I developed crippling headaches that took a peculiar form. Once a week I landed flat on my back in bed with a migraine. The pain was so intense I couldn't stand to have anyone near me. With the headache came vomiting, dry heaves, and horrible sounds I couldn't control. When the vomiting stopped, I went back to bed and lay still until the headache passed. After a good rest I felt energetic, as if none of this had ever happened.

After years of suffering, I finally began to understand what was happening to me. My tensions were continually being stuffed until I couldn't hold any more. The tension was then discharged through the headaches and violent vomiting. I had been carefully taught to flee conflict, not to fight.

A number of people have asked me, "Do you think there is one time when conditioning is more influential than others?"

My answer is "Definitely *yes*." Each child has sensitive, impressionable years when she is growing up. I believe these years vary from child to child.

The Dignified Prostitute

She had a nice, wholesome look about her, and she was a good mother to her son and daughter. No sacrifice was too great for them. She was also a prostitute.

I enjoyed working with Molly because she was very serious about counseling. She wanted to change in order to provide a better life for her children. She reminded me of the story of Dr. Jekyll and Mr. Hyde. I saw dramatic switches in her from one moment to the next. At night she may have slept in the gutter, but in my office I saw a side of her that was idealistic to the point of being "classy." Every now and then I noticed an air of sophistication and dignity slip through as she spoke. It puzzled me.

I consulted with an analyst about this case. He had been one of my instructors, and I liked his practical, earthy approach. When he reviewed Molly's case history, he said, "I want you to go back and get a new case history on your client. I have studied her life, but there is a missing link. Perhaps there is a period of her life she is leaving out because it's blocked from her memory. Go over her childhood year by year, and stop whenever she glosses over any period of time. As you explore, I think you'll find some answers."

I had already done what he requested, but I trusted his judgment. We started over, reviewing her earliest memories. Nothing was different until we hit the age of eight. She couldn't remember this year of her life.

We continued to explore, and eventually bits and pieces of the past came back to her. This is what she told me:

"My mother was a priest's mistress. He was a kind man, but he didn't like me living with my mother in the apartment he furnished for her, so he made arrangements and paid for me to go to a high-class boarding school in another city. I was there from the time I was eight until I turned ten. It was nice, but I rarely saw Mother.

"The school was owned and run by two elderly English ladies who took me under their wing and taught me the niceties of life. I'm not sure why, but they sort of protected me from the other girls. They were kind of like grandparents to me. I have happy memories of that school."

This was the missing link. These were significant years when her soul was indelibly imprinted. Why did she bury these few good memories when we had previously talked about her history? I can only believe what she told me. "Those were good years, but I hated the way Mother seduced a priest into supporting both of us."

What do I mean when I say Molly's soul was imprinted for life between the ages of eight and ten? I mean that during these years the experiences she had at the boarding school left a permanent impression on her. This accounted for the "classy" clues I picked up from time to time, in spite of her lifestyle as a prostitute.

I must tell you the end of Molly's story. She stayed in counseling with me for several years and, through a state rehabilitation funding program, earned a university degree. She then went on to become successful in a career.

The way we respond to stress may be either an automatic response or a consciously learned response that was imprinted in us while we interacted with power figures during childhood. My pattern of fleeing confrontation was not a result of religious training, although later this may have reinforced it. My flight response was due to the teachings I received from my British relatives who wanted me to become a proper young lady.

Something about childhood conditioning sounds fatalistic, doesn't it? Are we stuck with our programmed responses to tension? Are we to be victims of our past for life? Must we give up and say "I've always been this way, and that's the way it is"?

Of course not. As long as we live, change and growth are possible. I've had to make tremendous changes over the years to modify my flight-type personality. With each change came improved health and a higher quality of life.

As I've made choices to change my behavior, I've noticed my feelings and responses have changed, too.

That's what this book is all about. It's a book of hope that says, "Yes, you can change, you can undo the past." It's a book of tools that can turn life into a gift to be enjoyed rather than a sentence to be served. I can honestly say I'm not the same woman I was years ago, and life is more enjoyable. I've discovered some golden nuggets during my seventy-plus years of life. Now I'd like to pass them on to you. In the next chapter we'll look at storage pots and their relation to tension.

12

Our Storage Pot

I picked up the telephone in my office, and the caller identified himself as a lawyer. I knew his name and was curious
about the nature of the call. "I'm referring a young married
couple to you," he began, "because I want some feedback
about their marriage. They were married two years ago, and
every few months either the husband or the wife asks me
to begin divorce proceedings. I am concerned about them
because I think they have had a rough start from the beginning. I know their families, and they both come from stable
homes. My wife and I attended their wedding because we
are close friends of his family. If you think that the marriage
can't possibly make it, I will consider their latest request
for divorce, but I don't feel they've given each other a fair
chance. You do need to know that last week there was a
serious incident between them and they came to my office
immediately afterward."

I agreed to accept the referral, and the following week
the young wife, Sally, told me about her family. While she

was growing up they belonged to a large church, and all five children regularly attended services with their parents. They were active in the youth group and eagerly looked forward to being with their friends at church.

Sally's parents were very gentle to the point of being passive about many things. There was an unspoken rule in the family: keep peace at any price. Quarreling among the children was minimal, and Sally's parents were compatible. The children were taught that fighting was sinful and that they must love one another. If they did feel angry, they were to privately deal with it and ask forgiveness. Outbursts were not permitted.

Sally's mother didn't work outside the home and was laid back about housekeeping. Messes weren't important. She asked the kids to do the best they could cleaning their rooms and usually kept their doors closed. Home was a happy and relaxed place for Sally.

Marriage came earlier than Sally had planned, because of an unexpected pregnancy. Following the honeymoon she entered the work world in order to help support the family while her husband was in college. There were too many adjustments. She didn't know how to take care of an apartment; she hadn't learned to cook; her job responsibilities were changing; and now she was having to cope with a demanding toddler. Her biggest frustration, however, was the way her husband griped about everything she did. He constantly compared her with his mother, who was a perfectionistic housekeeper and top-notch cook who prepared everything from scratch.

"Can you please tell me about some of his complaints?" I said.

"Oh, that's easy. Take today, for instance. First thing this morning, before I had fixed a cup of coffee, he started in on me: 'Sally, there have been cobwebs in the family room for three weeks, and you've done nothing to get rid of those offensive things. And gravy spilled on the stovetop ten days ago and is still there. I don't know how you can be satisfied with such neglect! I never saw cobwebs in my parents' home.'

"I felt like saying, 'Well, fine, go home to your parents, then, if you like it there so much!' But I didn't. Like a good wife, I bit my tongue and didn't say a word." Sally mumbled something about believing wives should always be submissive and never fight back. I could see that within a few months of their wedding she had reached her limit for tolerating his criticism.

I still chuckle when I think about the first session I had with her husband, Ben. At the very beginning he looked me straight in the eye and said, "I want it perfectly clear that I don't like coming to a counselor. I don't believe in it, for one thing, and I don't need it."

"I am very glad you decided to come in," I replied. "Otherwise I have only one person's point of view. I cannot make an assessment without your help. It would be like working in the dark. If you'll help me, I'll be less likely to make a biased conclusion."

With a bit more calm in his voice, he said, "Well, I can understand your position."

"I'm grateful," I said, "because it makes my job easier. Your lawyer wants me to give him a report, and I don't want to pressure you into doing something you are firmly opposed to."

After a slight hesitation, he said, "Well, that's fine. I might as well talk, since I'm here. But I want it clear to you, we don't need a marriage counselor, because my wife is the sick one. She needs a psychiatrist. For what it's worth, I'll give you my side of the story.

"Sally is a disgusting housekeeper and refuses to take suggestions from me. When I point out things that need to be done at home, she deliberately ignores me. Just imagine; she leaves cobwebs hanging from the ceiling, even after she's been told they are there. It's a shame her mother never taught her how to keep house. My mother is appalled by her lack of order and cleanliness."

I interrupted his train of thought to find out more about the blowup his lawyer had mentioned. "Your attorney said there was an incident that happened in your home last week. Would you tell me about it?"

"Of course. It will show you why my wife needs a psychiatrist. I came home from school very tired. I work early mornings and then attend classes the rest of the day. When I walked in the front door, I went to the tiny hall closet to hang up my coat. It was disaster! Several pairs of Sally's spike heels were shoved into the closet, piled on top of one another. Her overcoat, which was halfway on the hanger, fell onto the floor, followed by her raincoat. How on earth can she expect her coats to stay hung when she throws them halfway on the hanger and then shoves them behind the door?

"Then I went into the kitchen, and baby John was wailing in his high chair. Sally was running around in her stocking feet, despite the fact that I have repeatedly told her it looks sloppy. I was angry and said, 'Sally, why don't you go upstairs and hang your clothes where there is more room in the closet, and take a few extra minutes to hang them up properly? I bought you a shoebag three months ago so you wouldn't have to clutter the floor with all your heels. I want you to use it, and while I'm here, would you please get the gravy off the back of the stove?'"

"How did Sally respond to you?" I asked.

This was the opportunity Ben had been waiting for to highlight Sally's mental problems. "Actually she never said a word. She just stood there and turned white. There wasn't much she could say, because she knew I was right."

"When did the fight happen that you referred to earlier?" I asked.

"I'm going to tell you right now. I went into the living room, and just when I was about to sit down, Sally rushed at me and literally attacked me, clawing my face. See the red marks?" he said.

I looked closely and did see one small red line down the right side of his face. Ben went on.

"I couldn't believe it. She was like a mad creature. I had to hold her down so she wouldn't keep hitting me. Then she sobbed and said she could not stand to live under the same roof with me one more day. Don't you see, Mrs. Lush? I was only trying to help her. She really needs a psychiatrist to help her stop those crazed outbursts against me."

The picture was coming into focus. The two individuals in this marriage were from totally different backgrounds. Sally's dad totally accepted his wife. Sally never saw fights or confrontations in her home. Their family motto was: peace at any price. The priorities in her family were extremely different from those in Ben's family.

The motto in Ben's home was: maintain high standards, no matter what the price. His mother was the perfect model and when Ben left things out of place, she yelled at him until he changed. Neatness quickly became a part of his life.

From the day this young couple walked down the aisle, the stage was set. Ben was critical. Sally played his doormat, all the while raging within. At the same time she had an angry toddler and a demanding job draining her energies. She had been conditioned as a child to put all her angry feelings into storage, but these feelings were highly flammable, and after a period of time could no longer be contained.

I'm afraid many women in America were conditioned to store their anger much like Sally. What happens when we consistently stuff our feelings inside? A story about Lyall will make my point.

Scraps in the Pot

Lyall came stomping into the kitchen, irate. "Why can't the folks in this house remember a few simple rules? I've been battling this garbage for years, and nobody listens. Look at this mess. There is food mixed with the papers and cans again. I have cut my fingers three times trying to separate this stuff. How many times have I asked you to put the plastic and the cans in one container, the burnable items in another, and the food scraps in a small pail? You know I bury the scraps in my compost. What else do I need to say before people get my message?"

I listened quietly and then responded. "Lyall, I'm sorry you're frustrated about the garbage, but it is impossible for me to enforce your system all the time. There are just too many grandchildren in and out of the house to keep track of it all."

"Surely they can learn a few simple rules!" he insisted.

"Why don't you try wearing your garden gloves so your hands won't get cut?" I asked.

Totally disgusted, Lyall said, "You know I hate those wretched things. Men in my day never wore garden gloves. They were only for women."

He was bound and determined to change the entire family rather than find another solution to his problem. The grandchildren never mastered his garbage procedure.

Lyall faithfully emptied the scrap pail by the sink every day and methodically burned the contents near where he would be planting new flowers. The neighbors hated his burning and burying, and murmured that they had seen a rat near the garbage pile, but nothing stopped him from contributing to the balance of nature.

Now why did Lyall bury the scraps *each* day? Most women can answer this in a second. Kitchen garbage stinks in two days. Fruit and vegetable peelings, scraps from plates, tea leaves, and leftover salad may seem harmless stuff, but the mixture ferments very quickly in a warm kitchen, and with fermentation comes a terrific odor that can penetrate the entire house.

The garbage pail in our kitchen reminds me of the anger we stuff into our own storage pots. Garbage must be processed daily. If it isn't, without any help from us, it rots and produces an ugly smell. The same is true for tension. When left unattended, it decays our soul and produces an ugliness that others are quick to detect.

I have found many sweet Christians with huge storage tanks deep in their psyches. Some have nice tight lids on their pail and don't notice their mounting problems, but eventually the odor seeps out and others catch wind of the rotting garbage inside. Others go to great lengths to protect their pail, keeping the lid on as long as possible, but it's only a matter of time before they find themselves in the middle of a breakdown.

Sally had a very large storage facility. Every day her emotions flared over the injustice of her husband's destructive nagging. She was angry about the early pregnancy and the horrendous demands of her job. Marriage wasn't supposed to be like this. She felt trapped in a prison without doors.

As a child Sally had never learned how to manage her angry feelings. She had learned anger was bad, and her rage frightened her. Not knowing what else to do, she simply threw her anger in the pot and jammed the lid shut.

It appeared to me that Sally was able to keep the lid on the pot for about three months at a time. Then came a blowout and a trip to the attorney. The tension during the last few months had become so unbearable that she finally went berserk. The lid exploded off the pail like Mount St. Helens' volcanic eruption, burning everything around her. She rushed at her husband, trying to hurt him, while screaming many words she later regretted.

I loved working with this young couple, because they were both willing to learn and neither of them truly wanted a divorce. Ben had to adjust much more than he had expected. Sally was not his mother, and she needed more help from him with the baby, as well as encouragement. Part of her anger came from her fears of being a failure as a wife and mother.

Sally needed to learn how to empty her garbage more frequently, so she felt more in control. Her tirades were ruining her marriage. As time passed, she learned to express her needs to Ben before a situation built up to explosive proportions. When criticism came, Sally began standing up for herself, saying something such as, "I have had a lousy day and I'm on edge. I'm not perfect, but I am trying to do a good job. Just give me a hug and tell me I'm okay. I wither up inside when you nag me."

Ben began to realize that he would rather have a wife who was warm and somewhat dependent in nature than a perfectionist wife who was more controlling, like his mother. A few years after we ended therapy, they called to announce the birth of their second son and assured me they were enjoying each other and looking forward to growing old together.

While growing up, many of us learned to react to tension in one of two ways: flight or fight. I considered Sally to be somewhat of a flight type, but not entirely, because she was aware of her feelings and stuck with the marriage. Some flight people deny their anger and totally avoid conflict, seeking peace at any price. Let's look more closely at the difference between flighters and fighters. See if you can figure out where you fit in.

13

Mrs. Flight

When I was working at the agency, I usually came home to an empty house. The children were involved in their after-school activities and Lyall had a very busy lecture schedule. Many times I was instantly irritated as I walked in the front door. Just one glance into the living room would start me simmering. Lyall would have changed his shoes and socks before leaving, and they would be dumped in the middle of the floor. His mail would be opened and left on the floor in disarray, along with sections of the newspaper.

When I left home in the morning, the house was tidy, but nine hours later every room I went into announced that Lyall had been there. I grew increasingly angry about the situation, and after several days asked him in a gentle way to pick up the things he had left on the floor. Nothing changed. I respectfully asked again. Nothing changed, except the level of my anger. It had moved from a level five to a level nine.

I noticed an odd thing about myself: when I came home, I began avoiding the living room altogether and stayed in the bedroom or kitchen.

About the same time this was going on, a supervisor at the agency began exploring some issues with me at the office. He said I never showed anger with anyone on staff, despite their deliberate efforts to provoke me. "This isn't meekness," he said, "it's weakness. You let the other therapists walk all over you." He also pointed to my fear of clients who displayed anger in session. Earlier I had requested that angry male clients be referred to someone else. He felt I suppressed my negative feelings too much and that I needed to quit running from them or I would never be able to help clients who suffered with anger problems.

This confrontation led to healing. All my life I had avoided anger. It was obvious my stoic British upbringing was adversely affecting me. I needed to stop avoiding and to start accepting anger as a natural part of life.

When I arrived home that night, I realized I had been avoiding the living room on the evenings Lyall was at the college. I didn't like anger, so I skirted the negative stimulus, pretending I didn't want to use the living room. I didn't consciously realize this until after my conversation with my supervisor at work. It was time to change.

That night I walked into the living room and allowed myself to be as angry as I wanted. Then I said to myself, "I'm going to tell Lyall to his face how angry I am. I'm tired of pretending. I work just as hard as he does. He needs to know how this is affecting me. This silent fuming has got to stop."

When he came home, I followed my plan. He mumbled something about my making a big deal out of an unimportant detail, but I wouldn't settle for that answer. I had played the doormat long enough, and it was harming me and our marriage. I restated my feelings, and Lyall got the point. The instant I gave attention to my feelings, I sensed relief, even before Lyall changed his habits. We both changed that day, and our love for each other grew because of it.

Before talking with my supervisor, I was a peacemaker. I never had the courage to be angry. I was frightened by the power of my own anger, so I ran away from it and others. My supervisor pointed out my need to change. The changes came about slowly, but they did come. My health improved, despite increased strains on the job. When I stopped avoiding and retreating, I had fewer headaches and more energy to manage difficult situations. The change in my work as a therapist was so marked that I was given a promotion.

Since then I've read many books on anger. I particularly like Dr. Theodore Rubin's work. He describes a certain kind of patient who is always tired. He feels this type of chronic fatigue comes from the way these people use their bodies to ward off anger or avoid showing any signs of anger. Generally these patients are in a chronic state of nervous and muscular tension. Their anger gets detoured to their muscles.[1]

I don't believe many flight people are aware of what is happening in their bodies. They have mastered the skill of repressing anger and avoiding people or situations that trigger anger. Avoidance is a key piece of the puzzle.

The sad result of this is that when we chronically repress anger, we also squelch other feelings, especially love. Many women I've counseled have spoken of feeling numb, or when asked, "How do you feel?" cannot answer. They have repressed their emotions so long that they are unable to distinguish one feeling from another. However, when they begin to empty their storage tanks, feelings of love and joy are restored. When we openly share our feelings in constructive ways, true love is never destroyed, it is strengthened.[2]

Still, being honest about our feelings is risky business and sometimes is not applauded. It's much easier to talk about a physical complaint than a negative emotion. At least, that's what Melody thought.

It was Tuesday night, and members of the home prayer and fellowship group had gathered for their weekly meeting. There were mostly couples present, except for a few young adults and Melody, a well-to-do widow who was respected in the church as a fine Sunday school teacher and assistant in women's ministries. Melody was always ready to pitch in whenever help was needed.

For several years Melody had suffered with headaches, but lately they had become incapacitating. She wondered if they were related to menopause. Her doctor couldn't find a medical cause and gave her a clean bill of health.

In general, Melody didn't feel well. Bad memories about her brother were seeping back into her mind. There were times when she felt as if she were going crazy. For years she had pushed these troublesome thoughts out of her mind. Part of her was jealous. She had always lived in her brother's shadow, never able to measure up to his brilliant academic career. Other horrible memories from grade-school years were locked inside, too.

This particular evening the leader of the group said, "Let's be different tonight. All year we pray for the needs of the church, our missionaries, and youth. Let's set aside tonight to pray for our most pressing personal concerns."

Melody wanted to talk about her bad dreams and intrusive thoughts about her brother, but she thought, *What would they do if they knew I hated my brother and have fantasized about killing him? They would never let me teach Sunday school again.*

Everyone went around the circle, sharing their prayer requests. When Melody's turn came, she found herself saying, "I'm so glad we are doing this tonight. I have had headaches for the last few years, but lately they have been much worse. I would covet your prayers."

Everyone pitied this poor suffering saint and eagerly helped carry her burden in prayer. The next Sunday her friends made a point of showing their concern and assured her they were faithfully praying for her.

Now imagine if Melody had answered a bit differently. Suppose she said, "Oh, I'm so glad we are doing this tonight. Some of you know I suffer with headaches. But none of you know that I hate my brother and that I think this may have something to do with my health problems. He has always fooled everyone with his charm, and my parents adore him. He's a leader in a successful church, and everyone loves him. But they don't know what he did to me. It's not fair. I hate him! If there was a way I could kill him and get away with it, I'd do it."

Many group leaders would be stunned and not know what to do. Some might interrupt her so she wouldn't go into more detail, saying, "Uh . . . Melody has a big problem. Would someone like to pray for her?" Chances are no one would volunteer and the leader would step in and pray something like, "Lord, You know all about Melody's problem, and we lay her concerns before You. Undertake in whatever way You see fit . . . Amen."

No doubt few would be able to concentrate after Melody's dramatic display of negative feelings. The following Sunday she would most likely be avoided at church. After all, who wants to be around someone who is fantasizing about killing her brother?

I think most of us are as guarded as Melody. Christian women in particular feel they must always be nice. It doesn't make any difference what denomination we are involved with, we probably share the same expectations about ourselves.

Why? Because when we fulfill the "good girl" image, we get secondary gain. In other words, we get strokes, pats on the back, promises of prayer, and comforting hugs. But when we are transparent about feelings of anger, the response we receive isn't so warm and fuzzy.

Women are discouraged from expressing their anger. We are taught to be nurturers, soothers, and peacemakers. Our job is to please, protect, and placate the world around us. Any direct expression of anger, especially anger at men, makes us look unladylike, unfeminine, less maternal, socially unattractive, or strident.[3] We pay a heavy price for a nice image. I believe peace at all costs is a price too high for most women. Let's look more closely at what else is involved with the "nice girl" image. Typical characteristics of flight folk are:

Strong desire to escape angry feelings	Introspection
Desire for peace at any price	Nonacceptance of feelings
Avoidance of conflict	Stifle feelings
Denial of anger	Large storage facilities
Rationalization of anger	Strong desire to please
Suppression	Morbid mental conversations
Repression	Inhibiting self-condemnation
Passive resistance (procrastination)	Increase of problems
Cause queasy vibrations in others	Avoidance of close relationships

Mrs. Flight as a Mother

Nine-year-old Johnny is walking down the sidewalk toward his home at 11:00 a.m. School isn't due to let out until

2:20. His mother is scrubbing the kitchen floor and notices him through the window. Immediately she feels tense. The first thought that comes to mind is, *Oh no. What has Johnny done now?*

Johnny wanders into the house. Mrs. Flight calls upon her powers of denial and concludes, *There are probably teacher conferences today and the kids were dismissed early.* When Johnny walks into the kitchen, Mrs. Flight blocks him from saying something that might make her feel more uptight by asking, "Johnny, you are home earlier than usual. Would you like a snack?"

"Okay, but I'm not real hungry," Johnny answers.

Both of them are silent for a while, and then Johnny can't hold it in any longer. He suddenly blurts out, "Mom, I didn't do anything. Tommy stole the lunch money out of the teacher's desk, but I got blamed." Then he tells a long rambling story about how he always gets blamed for everything. Finally he says, "My teacher wants you to call her."

Notice something: Mrs. Flight had a temporary flare-up of tension and then backed away from the fear that made her tense. She did this by denial.

Some new thoughts follow. *My Johnny wouldn't steal money. He never does anything like that at home.* Her mind continues to try to reduce the tension. *Oh, what if he did steal the money? I stole when I was his age, and I turned out all right. He's not a bad person, just a typical kid. All kids steal at least once in their life.* Now she feels some relief. She decides she won't make a big deal out of the incident by calling the school and asks her husband to talk to the teacher whenever it's convenient.

Do you see the pattern? Mrs. Flight did not want to face the problem. She denied the truth, saying there really wasn't a problem. She rationalized, saying she stole when she was young. She universalized, saying all kids steal, and she pro-crastinated by putting off the phone call and passing it on to her husband.

The shrill sound of the telephone interrupts her thoughts. "Hello, is this Mrs. Flight?" the caller asks. "This is Green Valley Elementary School. Our assistant principal needs to see you right away in his office. We are having a problem with your son John."

Now Mrs. Flight is shaking with anxiety. She feels trapped and cannot run from her problem any longer. Deep down she knows Johnny has many problems, but it took a crisis to make her face the facts.

Mrs. Flight and Marriage

Fern was nervous as she explained her family crisis. Two years before, they had moved from the city their children were born and raised in, to a small country town where they didn't know a single soul.

Her husband had always dreamed of owning a small busi-ness. For twenty-eight years he punched a time clock for a large firm in the city. After his birthday he decided he needed a change. They sold their lovely home, and the proceeds and private loans enabled them to move and start the small busi-ness. Fern was furious about the arrangement because her husband had no administrative or public relations experi-ence. He had had several conflicts with staff at his former place of employment.

When Fern came to see me, the business had been losing money for months. Worse yet, her husband had also drained her private inheritance fund, which she had reserved for their younger child's college education.

"Did you participate in the decision to move and start the new business?" I inquired.

"I tried to explain how I felt to Tony, but he blew up and said it was my job to support him and not to hinder his goals. He accused me of having no sense of adventure and no faith in him. I didn't know what to say after that. I've always wanted to be a supportive and submissive wife, but our life is awful. The kids hate the country, and we miss our old church. All I see in the future is bankruptcy."

Poor Fern. She was not only angry with her husband, she was angry with herself for being a doormat and not insisting on a feasibility study before buying the new business. Her husband acted impulsively, and she had not taken strong measures to stop him. Fern felt as if she had betrayed herself and her children.

Sometimes it takes a crisis to shake us out of flight mode. Fern's family forfeited everything, but today Fern doesn't see the losses as bad. She assumes half the responsibility for what happened and is now capable of stating her opinions, even in the face of opposition. That's a big switch from several years ago. Tony stopped playing the family dictator and gained a new sense of respect for Fern. He is grateful she stood by him when things were at their worst. Today when decisions are made, they do their best to reach an agreement before moving in a certain direction. Fern was forced to get a job outside the home to help support the family, but she doesn't regret the change. It has given her an opportunity to develop computer skills, which she in turn has passed on to her three children.

Fern and Tony lost everything they owned before change was realized. That's proof that change is difficult but always possible. As I listened to Fern talk, I knew we had something in common. Both of us wished we could be tougher, like

168

those who have mastered the "fight" response. However, kicking into fight mode creates its own set of challenges. In the next chapter you'll meet some people with raised fists who fought their way through life. They got results, but I'm not sure they found them rewarding.

14

Mrs. Fight

"I am so angry!" fired Agatha. "I received a memo from the head office accusing me of being sloppy with my paperwork."

"So did I," replied Betty.

"You did? Well, what are you going to do about it?" Agatha fumed.

Coolly and calmly, Betty answered, "Oh, think nothing of it. Everyone got one. I bet all the branch offices received the notices."

"Well, maybe," retorted Agatha, "but that notice was directed at me. That administrator hates me, and he is always trying to blame me for doing something wrong."

"But Agatha," Betty contested, "we all got the notices. Why are you taking this so personally? I don't finish my paperwork either until I absolutely have to meet the deadline. We all have room for improvement. I threw my memo in the wastebasket and just plan to try a little harder."

"Well, that might work for you, but I'm getting to the bottom of this. I'm going to fight back this time. That administrator has pushed me around one too many times. If need be, I'll take this up with the board of directors."

After her closing statement, Agatha stormed out of the office and went home to write a scorching letter of indignation to the administrator. He in turn read this to the rest of the supervisory staff and concluded, "I was thinking about giving Agatha more of a supervisory role, but now I don't think this would be wise. This letter is way out of line. All the branch office personnel received the reminder notice." Her letter was placed in her personnel file at headquarters. Consequently, Agatha was passed over for advancement positions while younger but more emotionally mature members of the business were favored.

Agatha was a fight person, and like most fight people she had difficulty accepting correction. Any criticism was taken as a personal attack. Fight people tend to impulsively attack in response and then complain about unfair discrimination. Actually, it was probably a good idea for Agatha to write the letter, but mailing it turned out to be a disaster. She and others who resort to the fight mode when they are tense share some things in common. These are the typical characteristics of those who are fighters:

Small storage facility

Discharge tension immediately

Act to reduce tension

Attack others

Aggressive

Aroused quickly

Touchy, irritable

Want immediate relief

Emotions feel out of control

Don't use reasoning and judgment

Attack before being attacked

Overly imaginative

Fear people are out to get them

| Frequent outbursts of temper | Destructive to self and others |
| Overly reactive | Reinforce own anger |

Mrs. Fight as a Mother

When nine-year-old Johnny came dawdling down the sidewalk from school three hours early, his mother became tense. Figuring he was in trouble, she immediately thought, *I hate this school. They always pick on my family just because we are poor. My kids get blamed for everything that goes wrong in that place. I'm not going to take it anymore. This time I'm fighting back. I'm sick and tired of that school harassing my kids.*

Even before Johnny walks in the front door, Mrs. Fight is in a high state of tension. Johnny had been this route before and knew his mother would jump to his defense.

As he enters the house, his mother says, "Johnny, are you in trouble?"

"Mom, I never did nothing," he says. "It was Tommy who did it."

"Tell me what happened," she demands.

"Tommy made me look in the teacher's desk, and then some money was gone. They all blamed me," explained Johnny.

In a burst of temper, Mrs. Fight yells, "This is the last time they are going to pick on us. Mark my words."

Mrs. Fight has a very small storage tank that can't possibly hold all the anger she feels. She must do something immediately for relief. She marches to the neighbor's house and bangs on the door. When the door swings open, she sharply scolds her neighbor. "Your Tommy has gotten my Johnny into trouble, and I will not allow my kid to catch the blame any longer."

Trying to reason with Mrs. Fight in this state of mind is impossible, but the neighbor tries. "I think Johnny has been stealing little things for a few months. I've heard children in the class complain about it. Maybe it would help for him to talk to the school counselor."

"How dare you say such things!" shouts Mrs. Fight. "You are part of a conspiracy at that rotten school. You're all out to make trouble for us."

Mrs. Fight stomps off and drives furiously to the school. Red in the face, she demands to see the principal. Johnny's file is sitting on his desk, and the principal is braced. He knows Mrs. Fight very well from her chronic complaints. Johnny is the last of her five children to attend the school.

Mrs. Fight storms into the principal's office. Quickly taking charge of the situation, he says, "Mrs. Fight, Johnny has been caught several times with things that belong to other children. He takes other children's belongings and then tries to give them away. Today he was caught rummaging through his teacher's desk, and the teacher reported some missing coins."

He goes on to describe his concerns and suggestions for helping Johnny, only to be rudely interrupted.

"You continually pick on Johnny. Everyone does, just because he is small and we're poor. If what you say is true, it is only because he gets rotten treatment at this school. I'm not going to stand for this anymore."

She roars out of the office and goes home. Guess who is going to get her bucket of anger next? Little Johnny. Seeing his mother lose control makes him feel more insecure, and the cycle continues. Nothing is faced, and nothing is changed. Johnny learns he must be more cunning and sneaky the next time he lifts something from one of the other children.

I realize I am being simplistic by labeling people as flighters or fighters. The truth is, we all react in a variety of ways, depending on the different situations that come our way. Yet most of us lean toward one habitual response. I don't recall meeting anyone who had both strong fight and flight tendencies. Usually there is a bent in one direction or the other.

Now I want to introduce you to some others. They know how to sit tight when they're tense. They don't keep peace at any price, nor do they carelessly spew their anger at others. See what you can learn from their examples.

15

Mrs. Sit Tight

Jean, I am disgusted with the way you are raising the children. Robin talks all the time and has no respect for anyone.
When you were young, you would not have dared to interrupt adults. Jean, you must do something about that child!

And David's mischievous naughtiness is the talk of the
town. You mark my word, Jean. David will end up delinquent
if he keeps on like this. His temper tantrums are despicable!
No child in my day ever acted that way. Do you or Lyall
ever give that child a good hard spanking? When we found
out the police showed up at your front door because he
was throwing stones at the neighbors' houses, we didn't
sleep a wink. The neighbors were in an uproar. He is only
3½! What is he going to do for thrills when he gets older?
Your dad and I feel he should not come to any more family
gatherings until he is better behaved. We are too old to put
up with his antics.

And another thing. Your children never have nice clothes.
Those two darling granddaughters of mine have never worn
a smocked frock. I always dressed you and Elaine in the best

attire. Your milkman says you have one of the biggest milk orders on his rounds. It is just plain silly to deprive your girls of silk dresses for all that milk!

And now Lyall is asking John to invest his savings in publishing Christian tracts and booklets! You shouldn't let your husband get himself and others involved in such crazy nonsense.

Mother's letter had not come at a good time. I was already physically and emotionally worn-out from nursing my baby and trying to manage a dreadfully prankish three-year-old boy and capricious five-year-old girl just starting school. Being cramped in our crowded little house during thermometer-breaking heat waves was almost unbearable.

I also lived in terror of the polio monster that was gobbling up both the young and old. An epidemic had swept through our state, killing families by the hundreds. Many children who did survive were crippled for life. School buildings were locked tight, and the children's public recreational gatherings were canceled for months. Many of my choices during those days were a matter of life and death.

Each morning when I rolled out of bed, it seemed the best I could do was hope for survival! I didn't have energy for long-term planning—no future goals, no dreams. Managing the day, one hour at a time, sapped all the strength I could muster. When Mother's letter arrived, it wasn't long before I was binging on self-pity.

All right, Mother. If my children are such a terrible disgrace for your family image, you need not ever see them again, I thought. *We will promptly drop out of your life. I've never achieved anything next to your brilliance, anyway. I know, I know. All my girlfriends married into money and I didn't. And now I have to make all my children's clothes. Oh, Mother! No matter what I do, I'll never please you.*

Somehow I gathered my senses together and ran next door to talk to my friend. "My mother would never write such a letter to me. How dreadful for you!" was her response. The support helped.

The rest of the day was a blur, but late into the evening, after the children were in bed, I turned to Psalm 37 for comfort. As in times past, God told me to wait, sit still, and not take action. I followed His advice, tore up the letter, and determined not to strike back. As the days went by, I did my best to dodge black moods by keeping incredibly busy.

Three weeks later another letter arrived. It was from my sister, who was preparing to get married. At the time she was living at home in the lonely hills with my parents, who had just retired. Her words caught me by surprise.

"Jean, Mother told me she wrote you a terribly stinky letter. She is very depressed over hurting you and fears you will never forgive her. Please write. Write anything! I have never seen her this down."

Shortly after receiving my sister's letter, I invited Mother to our home for lunch. During our meal, I learned she had been having heart trouble. In addition to her physical problems, all the fussing about the wedding was keeping her constantly agitated.

Several months before the wedding, Mother suffered angina pains. This affected her emotionally, and she unloaded her frustrations on me. She explained later that once the letter was mailed, she was very upset with herself for writing such cruelties. She actually sympathized with me about my burdens as a mother.

Over lunch Mother said, "Jean, you have always been the strong one in the family who was brave in the face of trouble. Please forgive me for all the nasty things I said. I need you."

From deep within my heart, I thanked God for instructing me to be silent and to wait for Him to work. Had I acted on my first flush of anger, I would have wounded my mother and lived with regrets the rest of my life. With her health problems, a retaliation on my part could have literally stopped her heart.

Often we are caught off guard when someone hurts us, and our immediate angry impulses are deadly vicious. These are times when we must pull back the reins on those wild urges and look to God for strength to sit tight until He shows us what to do next.

Mrs. Sit Tight as a Mother

It's 11:00 a.m. and Mrs. Sit Tight is scrubbing the kitchen floor. Out of the corner of her eye she sees Johnny, her son, walking toward the house. She is confused because school usually isn't dismissed until 2:20 p.m. Feeling anxious, she meets Johnny at the front door.

"Johnny, you are home early. Is there anything wrong?"

"Well, sorta," mumbles Johnny.

"Tell me all about it, and try not to leave anything out," she says.

Johnny tells a rambling story about how he was blamed for stealing, and his mother listens very carefully. Feeling even more anxious, she asks Johnny to tell her the story again. This time Johnny doesn't tell the story quite the same. The facts don't jive. Mrs. Sit Tight knows something is very wrong.

She decides she needs to talk to the neighbor next door and calls to ask permission to go over. After explaining Johnny's story to the neighbor, she listens very carefully to the information the neighbor offers. Apparently the neighbor's son and his friends have been talking of Johnny's petty thievery during the last several months.

The tension level continues to rise in Mrs. Sit Tight. She calls the school and makes an appointment to speak with the principal. An hour later she enters his office and says, "I know there is a serious problem with Johnny, and I am alarmed!"

The principal explains what he knows of Johnny's stealing and suggests ways to help him. He tells Mrs. Sit Tight that a social worker in the school district has volunteered her services.

By now, this mother's tension is beginning to ebb away. Johnny has a problem, but she is sensing relief from facing the problem. She's not running. She's not overreacting. She's gathering information from her neighbor and the school authorities and accepting the fact that her child needs help.

When her husband comes home, Mrs. Sit Tight is uneasy about the situation but is able to rationally communicate what happened during the day. Together they decide that Johnny must repay all the stolen money and anything else he took by using his birthday and Christmas money. They will also allow him to earn money at home doing extra chores. They both feel relief because they have done their best to responsibly take charge of the situation. The rest is up to Johnny.

I want you to notice some of the qualities that are unique to Johnny's mother in this story. Common characteristics of those who sit tight are:

Tend to be rational

Try to reason through conflicts

Focus on problem solving

Monitor and control their reactions

Acknowledge their anxiety

Wait before acting

Reduce tension before making decisions

Seek expert advice

Consult with others for input

I don't believe we are born with an innate ability to handle our tensions wisely, but I do believe we can learn through experience how to tame our tensions. We can resist being guided by impulsive emotions and learn to wait until reason can help us control our emotional responses. Eventually the use of reason will become more habitual, so there is less danger of responding with destructive outbursts. Looking back, I'm so thankful for the times I put a stop to effects of my outbursts and tore up letters I had written in indignation. There is one I remember particularly well.

My father was very excited about his retirement from public life. He was eager to carry out his plans on an old country farm he had inherited from his forefathers, but the farm was in an isolated area that separated my mother from all her friends and interests in town. She had never driven a car because when they lived close to town various means of transport were easily accessible.

I was furious with my father for insisting that he and Mother move to that old farm. I couldn't believe he expected my mother to enjoy that setting. She had never lived on a farm or in a country village.

I wrote a ghastly letter to him, denouncing him for worshiping that old farm and not being sensitive to Mother's needs. I thank the Lord for telling me to wait and sit tight. Eventually the letter landed in the garbage pail. Mother lived over twenty years on that farm and, thanks to the cool climate in that region, her health greatly improved. I shudder to think of the impact that nasty letter would have had on her, on him, and on me. Thank God I never had to find out.

Keeping the Lid on Tight

I recently read a book by Shirley Chisholm called *The Good Fight*. Though I don't support her political views, I have great admiration for her as a woman. It's hard for me to imagine the extreme pressures she endured in the role she chose. Shirley was the first black woman to make a serious effort to become president.

I particularly enjoyed a glimpse of her in action while she attended the annual exhibit of black achievements in Chicago. This is how she recapped the event:

> I went into the convention hall where I was to speak, along with Coretta King, at a workshop on women in politics. As I went into the hall, three or four black men came in at the same time. They were middle-aged and conservatively dressed. I took them for politicians.
>
> They saw me and one of them said loud enough for me to hear, "There she is, that little black matriarch who goes around messing things up."
>
> I was furious, but all I did was give them a hard stare.[1]

Now friends, that's self-control in action. Perhaps some of the greatest examples of self-control are found in the histories of outstanding black women who fought for reforms and achieved great accomplishments in the face of horrendous opposition. Think of Marian Anderson, the first black singer to perform at the Metropolitan Opera. An accomplished musician, this woman has sung at the White House and served as a delegate to the United Nations. Barbara Johnson was the first black congresswoman from the deep South. Coretta Scott King is the standard-bearer of the gospel of nonviolent silent change. So was Rosa Parks, the courageous black woman who refused to give up her bus seat to a white male.[2] These ladies mastered the art of speaking up when the time was right and sitting tight when it was in everybody's best interest. They knew when *to* and when *not to* lift the lid on their storage pots. I'm certain they endured painfully stressful times when these choices were next to impossible.

I've heard many women say they would love to be more self-controlled. They long to be more like Mrs. Sit Tight, but by nature they aren't. They are more like Mrs. Fight or Mrs. Flight. They say, "I don't know what I'm feeling" or "I'm constantly shooting off at the mouth."

I believe we have very little direct control over our spontaneous feelings, but we do have control over our behavior. Whereas we can change our feelings only to a certain degree, our behavior is still under the control of our will. Feelings can be changed by changing our behavior. What we do can change the way we feel.[3]

So what do we need to do? How can we change? Must there always be a crisis to shake us out of our dysfunctional patterns? Sometimes it takes a crisis, because some of us are more stuck in our ways than others. But not always. If we recognize our need and are willing to make the effort, we can change. Nonetheless, change won't come overnight, and it won't come without some good tools.

Those who sit tight know this—they used to be flighters or fighters, but they learned some basic skills for discharging their tension that now enable them to sit tight. What tricks do they have up their sleeves? We will discuss these ways of discharging tension in the chapters that follow.

SECRETS TO TAMING YOUR TENSIONS

16

Do Away with Disorder

A few years ago I received a letter from a radio listener who was very depressed. Apparently Patty's husband, Bob, believed money was to be saved, not spent. He didn't want her buying things for the house, even though he habitually bought expensive tools to tinker with in his garage. He felt these purchases were acceptable, but instructed Patty not to bring anything home from the store that wasn't edible or mechanical. She had memorized his standard line: "Money spent on things just for appearance's sake is wasteful and worldly."

If Bob and I were to share a pot of tea, I would say a few things to that young man. The poor guy needs some basic education. Beauty and a sense of order in your home are functional. They have a purpose and are not unnecessary luxuries. Creating beauty around us gives us a sense of accomplishment, charges us with energy, and reduces tension.

Beauty is not just for the rich and famous. It is right for everyone and fundamental to emotional health. You see, beauty creates energy.

Frank Lloyd Wright, one of America's celebrated archi-
tects, taught his students that beauty dissolves conflicts,
quiets us within, inspires us, creates a sense of happiness and
serenity, refreshes us, and consoles us in times of depression.
"Beauty," he added, "is not unnecessary or impractical." His
creative house designs prove he built what he preached.

I've talked with many clients and audiences about the importance of surrounding themselves with order and beauty.
Some have said, "But I'm so plain and ordinary. And besides,
I've got all the kids to take care of, and no money in the bud-
get for fancy things. Even if I had a few pennies to spend, I
wouldn't know how to decorate." If you are feeling this way,
this is a strong indication that you need some time out from
the daily pressures to recharge. It doesn't have to be costly.

Straightening up the house can give you an inexpensive
perk, too. Restore order. Tidy up. Put things away. Organize
those areas that are spilling over. Find a place for storing clutter. Better yet, let your garbage can do some work for you.
Toss out some of the stuff you haven't used for years. You'll
be amazed how this can bring a sense of calm to any room
of the house and make you feel better about yourself.

A recent family gathering left me feeling tired and depressed because several people had discussed some difficult
problems. In my usual way, I listened and absorbed many
of their worries. This morning I could not concentrate, so I
wandered around the house straightening things and making things more orderly. Gradually my tensions faded, and
here I sit with pen in hand.

It's strange: as humans we are restless, driven, and even
dysfunctional when we carry around a lot of tension. We
must find constructive outlets.

I've had a number of people ask me to define "sense of
order." I don't have a pat definition, because my sense of

order may be entirely different from yours. Each of us has different priorities, likes, and dislikes. In my house there are stacks of books in every room. This would drive some people crazy, but I love books and read several at a time. In my kitchen I keep certain utensils and appliances lined up on the counter for easy access. The blender, the juice maker, and the food processor are always at hand. This would look cluttered to some.

What constitutes your sense of order? Define it for yourself. Things don't have to be spotless to create peace, but they do need to be neat, according to your standards. Gloria Vanderbilt says it well: "I'm not talking about cleanliness . . . it's a sense of order that fills the house with a feeling of serenity and tranquility."[1] A well-known interior designer, Alexandra Stoddard, says: "When your home is in chaos, you become overwhelmed . . . you are affected by beauty and harmony. Clean up the outward turmoil, and feel the inner peace and grace . . . You get energy from beauty and it gives rich rewards."[2]

Beauty and order can create peace in the heart of children, as well. I remember learning this from dear Mrs. Frieze. One day she visited me at the Kings Garden dormitory, wanting to help with some improvements. Looking me straight in the eye, she said, "Mrs. Lush, I have never seen such shabby living conditions for teenage girls. I know many of the girls come from difficult backgrounds and suffer with depression. Something must be done to create more of an uplifting atmosphere for them."

I was overwhelmed by her generous offer but had no idea where to begin. The bedrooms seemed an impossible task, with their cold cement floors and old iron bunk beds. I think most of the furnishings had been there since the building was constructed in 1907 as a hospital and isolation unit.

Undoubtedly the beds, tables, and chairs had been army surplus. Rather undaunted by my concerns, she explained her plan.

"I have canvassed the entire building, and I want to start by redecorating the large living room. We will haul the old, broken-down furniture to the dump and replace it with sturdy ranch furniture, built especially to fit this room. We can also build in upholstered seating along the far wall, so there will be plenty of seats for the girls during dorm meetings."

As I said, I was thrilled with her offer, but overwhelmed, too. I had had a terrible time training the girls to responsibly care for their belongings. How would they treat the new furnishings? I shuddered to think of what the new room would look like after a year of use.

"Mrs. Frieze, I'm a bit dubious about the new furniture. These girls are pretty hard on this room. They are used to eating snacks in here and don't care what kind of a mess they leave behind."

"I have found," she replied, "that providing nice things for young people pays off. Once this room is redecorated, I think you will find them acting quite differently. They're messy because this room feels messy. I'm confident they'll respect their new furnishings."

Mrs. Frieze went to work. She used a beautiful color scheme of light green, cherry pink, and touches of silver in the wallpaper. The sturdy oak furniture was upholstered in a dark green fabric that was easy to clean. The transformation was amazing!

But even more amazing was the change in the girls. I wish you could have been there. After the room was completed, I never had to nag them to keep things tidy. The soothing impact of this living room affected their disposition and fostered some of the best behavior I had seen in years. Mrs. Frieze was right: beauty calms and restores.

Since the recent death of my husband, little tasks seem impossible to me. It's hard to make decisions. Direction and answers don't come quickly. A constant feeling of melancholy overwhelms me. Sometimes I wonder if there will ever again be joy or pleasure in this world for me. I feel like I'm a burden, and the future frightens me. As a therapist, I realize this is the nature of grief, but knowing that doesn't change my experience.

Recently I knew I needed to daily involve myself in something that would lift my spirits. The perennial English garden Lyall and I created together started to bloom. One afternoon while standing at the kitchen window that overlooks the garden, I sensed the flowers were there for me. I needed to allow myself to enjoy them, even though my beloved artist couldn't stand beside me, exulting in their beauty. Oh, how he loved that garden. I made a conscious decision that day to begin tending the garden again and to find joy in giving attention to the flowers we touched together for so many years.

Fall is here, now, and our collection of Japanese maple, vine maples, and dainty huckleberries are wild with color. The avenue of golden birch trees along our street glow by the light of the moon.

Sometimes I'm overcome with a rush of tears when I recall how Lyall loved this time of year, as only an artist can. All the while I'm learning that I can glory in the spectacular world of gold and pastel oranges on my own. Standing in my garden, I breathe deeply and soak in the beauty. Tension and fatigue ebb away, and I have the boost I need to go back inside and work again.

17

Diversions

Tom and Mary Brown were referred to me by their family doctor, who was puzzled by Mary's chronic fatigue. After many sophisticated tests, nothing could be medically pinpointed as the source of her problem. The doctor wanted me to investigate possible emotional or relational difficulties.

With his hands clasped in his lap, Tom began. "I just don't understand, Mrs. Lush. We have three beautiful children, and I love my wife very much. She is a full-time mother and takes pride in caring for her home and family. We love our church, and she has many friends. My job is steady, and my security with the company is good."

Shifting in his seat and then leaning forward, he continued. "But Mary is always tired. She sleeps over ten hours a night and still wakes up tired. Headaches bother her a lot, too. They aren't crippling, but she is rarely free of pain. Please help us get to the bottom of this. We need to know what to do."

Stepping into the conversation Mary added, "I know you've talked to my doctor, and everything Tom says is true. I don't know what else to tell you. I'm as confused as everyone else."

Slumping back in her seat, Mary stared at the floor.

"Perhaps you can start by telling me about your daily activities. Help me understand what you do during an average week," I replied, hoping Mary wouldn't withdraw from the conversation.

During the hour we spoke, I learned that Mary led an uneventful life. She had come from a good home and married young. The three boys arrived early, and she never worked outside her home. However, she was extremely busy seven days a week, serving others. Further on in our session, I commented, "Mary, you are a very giving person. You give to your husband, your boys, your church, your mother, and all your younger sisters. What do you like to do for yourself? What's fun for you? What are your needs?"

A blank stare swept over her face. It was as if I had just spoken in a foreign language.

"What do you mean? I'm a mother and a wife."

I tried to be more specific. "Do you have any hobbies apart from your family? Things you like to do for pure pleasure and enjoyment?"

Astonished, she said, "No! Do you know what shoes cost for growing boys? If I did things for myself, my children would suffer. I couldn't be that selfish."

I probed a bit more. "But Mary, what would you enjoy doing if you didn't have anyone else's needs to consider?"

"Well, that's a dumb question," she replied. "That's not reality!"

"True," I persisted, "but let's pretend for a moment." I waited.

"I don't like games and pretending. I don't need to do anything more than I'm doing now!"

She had a point. She didn't need to do more—she probably needed to do less, with more variety. I began to see that Mary was a very structured, duty-ridden individual who was not in touch with her own needs. She had spent her adult years tending to the needs of others at her own expense. I would need to catch her off guard if we were to get anywhere in therapy. Our conversation continued.

"Mary, tell me about your life as a young adult, before you married Tom."

"Well, after high school I planned to attend college. I had the wild idea of becoming a concert organist. I wanted to play gospel music at church," she replied.

"Did you learn to play the organ?" I asked.

"A little," she said with regret, "but after I had a few lessons we got married, and we were poor, and then I got pregnant right away."

"Did you ever think about those dreams again?"

"Not really. I didn't have money for lessons, or time, with the baby. Besides, it didn't seem right to pursue selfish interests that would take my attention away from my family."

Mary's physical problems made sense to me. She was all output and no input. What a wonderful way to become tired and headachy! I suspected that she was a perfectionist and never felt her work was done. After the hour was over, I requested a session alone with Tom.

The following week I asked Tom to describe Mary during their year of courtship.

"Well, in some ways she was very different. Full of fun, high-spirited, and always involved in a lot of activities. She enjoyed all kinds of music, and took organ lessons. After we were married, though, she never mentioned it again."

I had an opportunity and seized it. "Tom, I have a suggestion. I think Mary needs some creative outlets, and my hunch is that playing the organ would improve her health."

This seemed to create conflict in him. With a furrowed brow, he said, "Mrs. Lush, I want to do everything in my power to help Mary's health, but we cannot possibly afford an organ."

"Tom, when you need to pursue something as important as I suspect this is, you will find a way."

A few weeks following my appointment with Tom, a couple in their church announced they had an offer of a long-term position overseas. All their furniture was going into storage, but they needed a volunteer to keep their organ. The following week, that splendid organ sat in Tom and Mary's living room. Within a few days, Mary found an organ teacher who willingly exchanged music lessons for babysitting.

Six months later, Mary was energetic and headache free. In spite of all the household demands, she felt refreshed after eight hours sleep, and her work got done. I attribute her improved health to one hour a day at the organ. Playing the organ was an outlet for her tension. For Mary, this outlet was not a luxury; it was a necessity.

I travel across America, teaching stress-management strategies at conferences and retreats. Numerous audiences have shared creative diversions with me. The first remedy given in every crowd of women is, "Go shopping!" Of course, all the other women nod and applaud. Men usually mention some kind of sports activity. Here are some other diversionary tactics offered by men and women across the nation:

Read	Take a bubble bath
Play music	Have a makeup
Cook a gourmet dish	makeover

Get a massage

Call friends

Do some sort of craft

Attend classes at church

Go to school

Put duties on hold

Hunt antiques

Bargain hunt

Take a long walk

Go to the beach

Pour a cup of tea and just sit

Sleep

Take a long drive in the country

Exercise

Write in a journal

Cry good and hard

Clean closets and scrub floors

Write a long letter to a friend

Reach out to someone

Work in the flowerbeds

It really doesn't matter which of these you use, but it is important that you find some creative outlets to release your tensions. Diversions will make life more pleasant for you and for those around you.

The Emergency Call

I had just finished my dinner and was preparing to step onto the platform. The mental health agencies in our area had gathered for a lovely banquet. I was to address the group on the results of some research I had recently completed.

My thoughts were interrupted by a voice somewhere behind me. "Is Jean Lush here?" he said. "Her son is calling from the hospital. It is urgent she come to the phone."

Moments later I was talking with David.

"David, what is the matter? How did you find me?"

"Ma, Poppa is down here, and he is in the hospital," David replied.

"What do you mean he is down there? He can't be!" I retorted.

David didn't pay any attention to my irrational remark and continued. "Ma, I don't want to alarm you, but I am coming to Seattle to bring you down here to Pa."

"David, what is the matter with Poppa?" I shouted into the phone. "You must tell me right now. Is it serious? You are hiding something from me. Is he all right?"

"No, Ma, Poppa is not all right. He may be having a heart attack. He has suffered a terrible blow in his business and has kept it from you. I can't talk about it now. Just wait for me there, and I will come right away. Give me the address," he said sternly.

I gave him the address, and the phone went dead. I was numb and white with terror as I returned to my seat. I knew Lyall had been thinking about driving down to David's to discuss an art show, but I didn't know he had already left town. I had been gone since early in the morning. Apparently he started his drive south after I left home.

Somehow I climbed up onto the platform and presented my research on 150 married couples who answered the question: What do husbands say are their greatest dissatisfactions in marriage?

David arrived before the program was over and told me I had to come dressed as I was. It was imperative we get to the hospital immediately. He was direct and to the point. "Ma, Pa is going to be all right, but we were there to help him just in the nick of time. He is dreading your visit because he doesn't want to tell you about a business problem he has been hiding."

"I don't understand," I cried. "What do you mean, business problem?"

"Ma, Poppa has been sued by a business colleague, and he may be involved in a court case. It has something to do with a complicated art issue I don't fully understand."

"Oh, David!" I moaned. "I had no idea Pa was under such strain. He hasn't mentioned a word of this to me. I noticed he was more quiet and remote lately, but this. . . ."

My voice trailed off as I looked into the distance, worried about Lyall and fearing what lay ahead of us.

The visit with Lyall was difficult for both of us. He was in no condition to discuss the legal battle. He felt like a complete failure. During all our years of marriage, Lyall had always protected me from financial concerns. His father and successful older brothers never burdened their wives with business matters, and he followed suit.

As the days passed, Lyall's heart condition improved rapidly, and tests revealed there was no damage, but he was very depressed. A black cloud of despair overshadowed him all the time, making everything burdensome. The most simple and mundane tasks seemed monumental.

The doctors told me his depression was a result of the drugs he was being treated with and his adjustment would take time. I had never seen Lyall like this before. He was such a positive, happy, and lighthearted person. I was living with a different man. Now he snapped at everyone, especially me, had no tolerance for frustration, and lashed out unpredictably.

When he first came home from the hospital, I took all my vacation time to be with him. The depression continued. One morning I had a brainstorm. Lyall always loved a change of scenery. I suggested we take the long ferry ride over to Victoria, Canada. This was one of his favorite spots, and I thought it might give him a boost. We had a nice time together, and his mind was diverted, but things seemed to be much the same when we got home.

I became more ambitious. Next I decided to risk the long drive to Banff, in the Canadian Rockies. We had little money to spend, but I sensed it was absolutely necessary we get away. Since it was still early in the year, we figured we could probably find a cheap hotel. Off we went.

Our time away was different from any other vacation we had taken together. We made a pact that we would put our troubles on hold. We agreed not to converse about our problems or even make passing reference to them. Instead we allowed our minds to be completely immersed in the magnificence of the towering Rockies. We aggressively snatched all the happiness we could during those six short days. Pretending we didn't have a care in the world, we entered fully into the joy of the occasion. We played and acted like kids discovering the wonders of the world for the very first time.

The diversion was enormously refreshing, but I sensed Lyall's despair was affecting him not only emotionally, but also spiritually. For the first time since his dramatic conversion many years before, Lyall was spiritually depressed.

I didn't know what else to do to help Lyall. It seemed my efforts weren't as effective as I had hoped. In desperation I whispered, "Lord, please help Lyall. Please, God. Give him hope."

During the last few hours of our stay in Banff, while we were surrounded by the awesome splendor of the snow-capped mountains, Lyall laid his fragile wounded life in God's hands. I remember his prayer as if it were yesterday.

"Oh, God! I don't know what to do. Everything has gone wrong. I don't have any answers. I don't know what is ahead of us. But, God, whatever happens, I will depend utterly on

You to show us the way. I will rest in You and face the months ahead, one day at a time."

That morning Lyall had read the book of Colossians. The wonderful truths in that book had come alive in him: "He is before all things, and in him all things hold together. . . . Let the peace of Christ rule in your hearts. . . . Set your minds on things above, not on earthly things" (Col. 1:17; 3:15; 3:2). Toward the end of our stay in the Rockies, Lyall had a deeply spiritual experience that left him a changed man. From that time forward, he began to sleep peacefully. His renewed trust in God obviously had a positive effect on his health.

As we were driving home from Banff, Lyall told me he was ready to face his legal problems. The dark depression was left in the mountains behind us and never returned during the following year of crushing stress.

It is a well-known fact among the medical profession that our state of mind has an enormous effect on our bodies. Dr. Redford Williams, a specialist in heart research, discusses the impact of chronic stress: "If we are to reduce heart disease, experts have to look at the psychological realm. Others have already noticed the impact of the mind and emotions on the body. Mental worry, severe grief, or a sudden shock may precede directly the onset of heart attacks."[1]

Dr. Archibald Hart, another stress-management expert, points to the necessity of diverting the mind. He says we must aggressively work to untrouble our minds and force our minds away from the problems at hand. If we want to reduce our stress, we must learn how to divert our thoughts to less troublesome matters.[2]

When I shared the importance of diversions with men and women in the counseling office, some balked and said the idea was ridiculous. "It isn't honest," they argued. "I wouldn't be living in reality. Besides, I'm too responsible to run away from my problems. I can't rest until I know the problem is solved."

Unfortunately these individuals end up wrestling with problems much longer than people who give themselves permission to be diverted for short periods of time. Solutions come slower and with greater difficulty. Locking on to problems until they're solved actually cripples our ability to find solutions and leaves us exhausted. Answers are more easily detected by an open, peaceful mind, rather than one that is hypervigilant and anxious.

Lyall and I found this to be true. By the way, he and I survived that difficult year that followed his time in the hospital. His terrible legal problems were miraculously solved without a court battle, and we were most grateful that Lyall never again suffered heart problems.

The week we spent in the Canadian Rockies taught me a lesson I've never forgotten: diversions are a gift we can give ourselves and others who are under chronic stress. Purposely untroubling the mind isn't a sign of irresponsibility. It's a smart choice that opens the door to restoration and spiritual renewal. Diversions quiet our heart so we can hear God and receive the direction and encouragement we need for the road ahead. I think the psalmist understood this when he penned the words: "He makes me lie down in green pastures, he leads me beside quiet waters, he restores my soul" (Ps. 23:2–3).

Defusing

"That will be seventy-eight dollars, Mrs. Lush," the man said as he closed his toolbox.

What? Seventy-eight dollars! I thought at the sound of his words.

I was outraged! How dare he charge me such a hideous fee for such a little job? All he did was remove two blinds from the inside of my skylight. It took him barely five minutes!

After he left, I wandered around the house like an angry animal trapped in a cage. I was mad and felt compelled to get out. *I need to go for a fast walk or dig up the garden,* I thought. Unfortunately, the cold, heavy rain pelting against my kitchen window reminded me that being outside wasn't a good idea. It was as if my body was looking for a way to get rid of my frenzy. I needed some sort of vigorous activity that would literally push the tension out of me, so I could concentrate and have peace.

Things got worse. The next day his secretary called and demanded that I pay the bill immediately. Hearing her cold, harsh words, "It's not my problem the fee is so high for a five-minute job," was like pouring gasoline on my fire. I nearly exploded.

Why can't people be more sympathetic? I thought. *Don't they know I've just lost my husband? Lyall could do the job if he were here. And all the bills. . . .* I found myself despairing as the tensions escalated. Fortunately I held my tongue until hanging up the phone. Then my kitchen walls caught the flack. This was a time when talking about the situation didn't seem to help. I needed some kind of physical activity to defuse my anger.

I remember when I first discovered the power of defusion. Years ago Carol came to me for counseling. She was having problems in her marriage and wanted to learn how to control her temper. During therapy it became evident to me that she was bitter toward her father, who had teased and belittled her while she was growing up. She married hoping her husband would indulge her with love and that the emotional abuse from the past would be left behind.

Her husband was a quiet, reserved man who also felt emotionally deprived. He didn't know how to show love or affection, although he did have deep feelings for Carol. Still Carol didn't know he cared, so she provoked him in silly ways to get his attention. When he didn't show affection, she tried making him mad. She was slowly ruining her marriage without realizing what she was doing.

Unexpectedly they were given a lovely vacation. I said to Carol, "Now is the time to aggressively make some changes. Put forth a supreme effort to control your outbursts and try to find some creative ways to show your husband some affection."

When she returned several weeks later, she was pleased by the improvement in their relationship and said she had not screamed once during the vacation. However, she also told me that she was waking up every morning with a headache that lasted through the day.

That afternoon I realized Carol had simply exchanged one destructive way of dealing with her anger for another. She went from externalizing her fiery feelings to internalizing them. She needed a healthy outlet to vent that anger.

I made a suggestion. "Carol, I want you to try something this week. Continue to control your outbursts, but add something to this assignment. Make time in your schedule for daily physical exercise. Mow your lawn, walk, garden, or do something that makes you perspire and gets your blood moving."

The change was extreme. Carol could not wipe away her abusive past. She couldn't change her husband; but she could make some choices that improved her physical and emotional health. During the next week her headaches completely disappeared. As time passed, there was such a marked improvement in her marriage that she and her husband were considered eligible to adopt a baby. Previously they had been refused because of the obvious conflicts between them.

Exercise is one way to push tension out of our bodies, but there is another way, too. Identifying with something aggressive also diffuses tension. I know many frustrated wives who complain about their husbands being addicted to television programs filled with action and violence. I can understand this, because the payoffs are substantial. People with sedentary jobs vicariously identify with the action and emotion on the screen, and this defuses stress. Of course, moderation is far better than addiction. Anything in excess will add to our problems and wear on our relationships.

Even Queen Elizabeth watched the television series "Kojak" whenever she had a quiet evening. You may think this is a weird program for royalty. Perhaps. But it's very functional for an overworked lady whose suppressed feelings needed to be discharged.

Dillydallying

When I was a youngster in Australia, I said to my best friends, "Whatcha doing today?" They replied, "Ah, nothing much. Just mucking about and dillydallying around. Come on over when you've finished your chores."

It always thrilled me to hear those words. Looking forward to the sheer fun and freedom of dillydallying never failed to help me finish my chores in a hurry. I couldn't wait to play without duties or worries to concern me. Sometimes we played hopscotch, skipped rope, painted, or colored pictures. If we wanted a bit more adventure, we climbed trees to hunt for bird eggs or built campfires and fried "chips" (potatoes). Those were the good old days.

It was wonderful growing up in an Australian country town. The scrub nearby smelled of sweet wildflowers. Orchids filled the air with their beautiful perfume. I loved dashing about through the fields, hunting lizards and snakes, always careful not to get too close to the poisonous critters.

Then there were the Saturday excursions to the big swamps. We swam and played hard until the last little bit of sun set in the west. I now realize those swamps were alive with tiger snakes, but I guess we made enough noise with our laughter and fun to scare them off. Today I shudder to think that I swam in the treacherous currents of that big river, but life was charming as we dillydallied without a care in the world.

I have concluded that we never really grow up. Oh, we age and mature, but there is always a little child in us that needs to play and get lost in fun. The older I have gotten, the more I've felt pressured to make time count, to be goal oriented, and to involve myself in things that are meaningful.

I think most of us are under too much stress, and we need to bring balance to our lives through play. Even some of our relaxation becomes too planned and goal oriented. Our determination to use free time "wisely" creates stress of a different kind. Dillydallying is good for the soul.

Many years ago Lyall and I traveled to England shortly after I had had a hysterectomy. Still in pain when Lyall suggested the trip, I said, "Climbing four flights of stairs in a cheap London boardinghouse is not my idea of a vacation!" We went anyway and wasted the days away. We visited the art galleries and strolled the streets. There were no phones to answer, no schedules to meet. We catered to our whims, coming and going as we liked. Even though walking was painful, I did find England refreshing.

I know of another way to dillydally anytime or anyplace. I call it mental play; others refer to it as daydreaming.

Daydreaming

Successful stress managers have the ability to create for themselves periodic islands of peace. Whether we are behind our desk at work or ironing six baskets of laundry, daydreaming can break the cycle of chronic tension. On your island of peace you can build the residence of your dreams—a castle, a log cabin, or a Victorian house. Perhaps it's a little farm like the one where you spent summers with your grandparents. It can be as plush as a modern penthouse flat or as simple as a little grass hut.

Imagine your house on a tiny island far from all your cares and responsibilities. There is a boat at the water's edge waiting to whisk you away to paradise. As you step into the boat, your worries magically disappear. Your wealth and resources are unlimited. The people on the island are totally compatible with you. Whatever you want is delivered at the snap of your finger.

This isn't rational, you say! Of course not, but it's beneficial.

I have an island of peace where I can pick fresh vine-ripened strawberries and lush golden papayas every day. There I can have my fill of tropical salads made with exotic fruits from around the world.

When I'm feeling noble, I go to my palace bedroom suite in London. After a brisk, refreshing walk around the palace gardens and a perfumed bath, an authentic English breakfast is served to me by maids and butlers.

Sometimes I lay by a lovely unspoiled lake on the palace grounds, watching swans gracefully glide across mirrored waters. I can instantly visit Lake Louise in the Canadian Rockies or the Lake District in England. Daydreams take me east in the fall, to brilliant colors dancing in the trees, and on to a Swiss chalet where I sit by a crackling fire, viewing the majestic Alps outside my window.

There is another imagination game I love. One of the greatest antique centers in the northwest, called Snohomish, is thirty minutes from my home. Set in a restored old historic town, one unique four-story building features specialized collectibles.

When I'm following game rules, I never say, "I'd love to buy that item, but I can't afford it." Instead I say, "Oh my! Look at this gorgeous piece. I rather like it. I think I'll have it." Then I make a list of everything I want for my English cottage. I nearly drool over the old Limoges china and the cranberry glass. As I peruse the antique cutlery with pearl handles, I list exactly which pieces I want for my collection. Remember, this has no relation to what I can actually afford—it's simply a fantasy created for my own enjoyment.

Other members of my family have great fun playing along with me. Sometimes even Lyall chimed in and added to the fantasy. He had a knack for picking out some of the most unusual artsy collectibles. We shared a lot of laughs in that old antique shop.

A simple five-minute imaginary game can bring emotional relief. Some people may call this splitting, or an irresponsible way to check out of reality. I call it dillydallying or mental play for the purpose of reducing tension. When an immediate change in routine or a luxury vacation isn't possible, we can always use our imaginations to create an island of peace.

If it's hard for you to daydream, hang around children and ask them to tell you stories. They are experts at using their imagination. Boys and girls freely use fantasy to cope with the pressures of life. Unfortunately, many of us take ourselves much too seriously and, in the name of maturity and responsibility, work too hard. May I encourage you? Take time for make-believe. Abandon yourself in play. I think God gives us an imagination for a reason. Christ knows the pressures we endure. Perhaps this is one reason He encourages us to "become as little children."

Distractions

"How have you tolerated so many years of hearing so many problems from so many people?" It's a question I frequently hear, and it's usually followed by something like, "I'd go berserk listening to people talk about their problems day after day!"

It's true, my life has been full of stress, in more ways than one. I didn't choose this kind of life, yet I wouldn't change it even if I could. By nature I am a homebody. I have never needed entertainment to keep me happy, and I really don't care to travel. In fact, traveling by air terrified me most of my life. It was only after I was in my seventies that I boarded a plane without someone with me for moral support. It takes a special person to deal with my anxieties on an airplane. My granddaughter Heather recalls one of her trips with me:

Nana and I were on our way to southern California for a broadcast with Dr. James Dobson on "Focus on the Family." I made sure our plane reservations to and from Los Angeles were on Boeing planes. She was convinced they were the only safe planes in the air. Shortly before Nana completed her interviews, my husband, Grady, called, asking me to catch an earlier flight home because visitors were coming into town.

I arranged for an earlier flight, but no Boeing planes were available. I knew Nana would be terrified getting on a plane made by another manufacturer, so I did everything in my power not to let her notice.

Boarding the plane, I stayed immediately in front of Nana to block her vision while we climbed the long staircase to the door. After seating Nana, I walked to the front of the plane, searching for a stewardess. "Please don't announce the type of plane we're on," I pleaded. "My grandmother will freak out if she hears the manufacturer's name. She's neurotic about flying on certain planes," I explained.

The stewardess told me it was company policy to make three announcements during the trip, all of which included the manufacturer's name. Exasperated, I returned to my seat, knowing I would have to distract Nana's attention from those announcements.

Every time I hear Heather tell this story, I giggle like a schoolgirl, because I had no idea what was going on. I couldn't understand why she was so talkative and animated during the trip. I thought perhaps she was excited about her husband meeting us at the airport or anxious about their visitors coming to town.

During each announcement, Heather talked to me so fast and furiously that I never once heard anything the stewardess said. Nor did I struggle with my usual panic. The power of distraction was at work.

We need distractions to relieve tension. I have several that I depend on consistently. When I go to bed, I read plant catalogs and books or magazines that display beautiful homes and furnishings. This is very different from the stimulating investigative reading I do when I am researching. My purpose at bedtime is to wind down and reduce tension.

During the day, a few minutes in my English cottage garden quiets my spirit and rests my mind. I find I need to do this several times a day when I am working hard on certain projects.

I love to grow climbing roses. In the midst of my studies I sometimes stop and take a few minutes to prune them or tie them into a new position. When the thought first crosses my mind, I argue with myself, saying I must keep working in order to meet my deadline. Now I'm discovering it is never a waste of time to distract the mind for a few minutes. This actually enhances productivity.

I also read about remarkable women of courage who contributed something unique to the world. A couple of years ago I was entranced with the accounts of Jenny Churchill's eventful life. Each time I opened the book that told of her marriage and various activities, I was transported into her world, forgetting everything else around me.

The private life of Queen Victoria intrigues me, too. This tiny woman was amazing. She bore many children, suffered terribly with premenstrual tension, and yet developed and ruled an empire for sixty years.

The things that distract me may not work for you. Lyall used to laugh at my bedtime reading selection. He much preferred a good devotional or philosophy textbook. My father, who was a public figure in Australia, loved the novels of Sir Walter Scott and algebra textbooks before going to sleep. Imagine that! Algebra textbooks!

I have a brilliant counselor friend who has had one of the longest active professional lives I have ever known. She reads mystery stories before going to sleep. Now this would release adrenaline into my bloodstream and keep me awake nights, but for her it reduces tension.

Think about it: what distractions can you build into your day?

Most recently I have found that distractions have allowed me to survive. Being with Lyall through his twelve surgeries and death felt like more than I could endure. For over two years, very heavy weights hung on a very thin wire. The worry, the grief, and the terrible sense of loss severely tested my limits.

What kept that thin wire from snapping? God's supernatural help and the tools you are reading about in this book. Time and again I've needed to firmly tell myself, "Jean, you must distract yourself when grief is killing you." I frankly think grief would have killed me, had the distractions not been there, but they were, and today there's even a bit of slack in the wire.

Debriefing

"Please clear your lunch hour for me," Jane whispered urgently. "I've got to talk!" I knew her well, and it was obvious something was bothering her.

A while later we sat across from each other in a local restaurant and ordered a salad. I waited. The moment the waitress left our table, Jane said, "I'm furious with my family! I can't believe what they did to me this weekend! Saturday morning John left for his men's fellowship breakfast before I woke up. He was gone all day! He knew I needed his help with all the household duties, but did he offer? No! He went with his friends to see a piece of vacation property they had recently bought. The boys bailed out on me, too! They left early for a scouting activity. There I was, with everyone's messes staring me in the face. I work longer hours than any of them. It's not fair that I have to do all their work and mine, too."

I could tell this had been going on for quite some time. This Saturday wasn't the first occasion Jane had been left with all the family chores. I kept quiet and listened, absorbing her tension.

She continued. "I've tried everything! I've hinted, I've reminded them with notes. Nothing works. I'm going to have to do something drastic to make my point. I can't counsel and carry the entire workload at home, too."

"What do you plan to do?" I asked carefully.

"I'm going to teach them a lesson they will never forget. They deserve some punishment for the way they have neglected me," she said. "I'm going to leave home and go to a motel. I'll stay there until they realize what I am going through."

Now this was not the Jane I knew. As a therapist she was skilled at managing her anger, but the weekend ordeal had tapped her limits. As her friend, I wanted to help her consider some other options.

"Jane, what else could you do to help your family understand your needs?"

"Oh, I don't know," she muttered with exasperation. After a few minutes of silence, she came up with an alternate plan. "I guess I could call a family meeting. They need to know I'm overloaded and need help." With a deep sigh she concluded, "There's got to be a solution. Maybe we can find it together."

There was some relief in her voice this time.

Toward the end of the week I asked Jane how things had turned out at home. She was pleased to share the results. "We all realized that we had drifted into a rut. The more I did, the less they pitched in. We made a list of all the chores and divided them among the family. We also decided to do some chores on weekdays so everything isn't left for the weekend."

I was impressed with the family's solution. More importantly, notice that Jane's skillful management of her problem was closely related to the time we shared over lunch. Jane had debriefed her anger the day before their family meeting, which enabled her to constructively solve the problem with her family.

Everyone needs at least one close friend they can absolutely trust when they are on overload. This is usually easier for women than for men. It is a matter of common knowledge that men do not have as many close friends as women.[3] Men's relationships are marked by shared activities. They tend to *do* rather than *be* together. Women's friendships more naturally rest on shared intimacies, self-revelation, nurturing, and emotional support.[4]

My husband used to remind me that it is difficult for men to be transparent. By nature men are more careful and guarded when they discuss themselves. During their childhood years, few men had male role models who displayed openness and vulnerability. If you study little boys, you'll often find them laughing at any exposure of intimate feelings. Their explanation? That's girls' stuff. Women are different.

I belong to a support group that has been meeting every Thursday evening since 1977. We call this group This Sisterhood. We are a diverse group made up of young and old, rich and poor, uneducated and highly educated. However, we have this in common: a love of God and a commitment to one another as women. Every Thursday evening we listen to one another's burdens, heartaches, joys, and victories. When several of us lost our husbands during recent years, we didn't hold back our sorrows from one another. This was one safe place we didn't need to pretend to be strong. Tears were understood; so was laughter. We have had hilarious times sharing stories about our children and grandchildren while reliving early life experiences.

I cannot tell you how much this group has helped me cope with stress over the years, especially recently. They were there when Lyall and I were told that he would need a serious operation. They continued to be there during the twelve operations that followed. Each time Lyall and I faced those surgeries, my hopes clung to the fragile chance that this time the operation would be successful and his life would be spared. My friends were very patient and tender, perhaps knowing all along that nothing was going to spare that very special man.

They were there to understand the awful melancholy that followed Lyall's death. They allowed me the freedom to share my deepest hurts. They didn't act shocked when I told them I didn't want to go on living for fear I'd become a burden to my family and everyone else. Talking has helped me to let go of Lyall a little at a time. I'm still in process.

As I sit here in my writing den, I can see the beautiful birch trees outside my window. Their brilliant colors are on full display with the coming of fall. It's peaceful now, but on stormy days fierce winds tear at the lovely leaves and whip the branches to and fro. Yet the trees continue to stand.

After Lyall's death, painful feelings stormed inside me, tearing down my desire to live, clouding my vision for God's call on my life, and smashing my hopes of ever feeling joy again. During this most difficult time, I realized that debriefing wasn't an option. If I was to go on living, it was a must. Thanks to some listening ears, I'm still standing in spite of the storm, and joy is coming back in bits and pieces.

18

More Ways to Discharge Your Tension

Diversify Your Interests

There is a hackneyed witticism that says, "Avoid women who are caught up in a diet, caught up in a divorce, or caught up in a doctoral program."

What do these women have in common? The word I would choose is *obsession*. They are intensely focused, unable to relax, stressed-out all the time—and with good reason. Their challenges are pervasive. They are constantly faced with pressures that have no end. I think many of us can identify with their dilemma during certain periods of life.

Some neighbors, Harry and Anna, were married for about sixteen years when the marriage slowly began to disintegrate. Harry was distraught and wanted desperately to save the marriage. From morning to night, Harry tried to figure out ways to help the marriage. Nothing else mattered.

When he came to talk with me, Harry was utterly exhausted. He and Anna were living separately, but they went to dinner together one evening a week. Harry was frustrated because he didn't see any positive changes in the relationship. If anything, he sensed more coolness coming from Anna. No matter what he tried, nothing helped, and he was downright confused.

So was I. In the majority of cases when a good man tries to be a better husband, usually he reaps good results. The opposite was true for Harry—he was losing ground.

One afternoon I said, "Harry, it seems to me you live from one dinner date with Anna to the next. What goes on when you and Anna get together? Are you both enjoying these times?"

I understood the nature of the problem from his response.

"Jean, don't play games or skirt issues. Our dinner date is the only chance we have to discuss our problems. How else are we going to reconcile if we don't talk honestly about the resentments between us? She needs to see the light."

Here was an opportunity for me to be direct. I got straight to the point.

"Harry, you and Anna are my friends, and I don't want to see your family torn apart. I know you are upset that this has been hard on your children. I must be frank with you. You are missing the only chance you have to reconcile by focusing on problems when you take Anna to dinner. I'd like you to steer the focus of the evening onto things that are pleasant and happy. Pretend you are courting. Strive to make a wonderful impression on her. You've tried the other approach, and it has gotten you nowhere. This is another option that might turn the tide that is threatening to drown your family."

Harry looked at me with a puzzled frown and said, "I don't understand you, Jean! I'm sick with worry about our marriage, and you're asking me to pretend nothing is wrong. I can't play games. I don't see how we can have fun together until we settle our differences."

I persisted with my suggestion in a number of different ways, but to no avail. You can probably guess the outcome. It wasn't long before their divorce was final. Some contrast at this crucial point in time might have revitalized their relationship and awakened a spark of interest in Anna, but it never happened.

Years ago, John Stuart Mill said, "The mind does more by frequently returning to a difficult problem than by sticking to it without interruption."[1] People refer to vacations as being a good "change of pace" or contrast to their usual routine. Many who live in the Northwest, with our dreary alpine winters, find a haven in the Hawaiian sunshine. One or two weeks away changes their outlook on life. Even tourists who jet from one attraction to the next come home rejuvenated. The pace didn't refresh them, but the diversity did.

My son, David, is a physician, and he has spent much of his life dealing with emergencies in a country hospital. After a long night delivering babies, he comes home exhausted. Then instead of heading straight to bed, he tinkers around in the garage with messy old car engines. This is in total contrast to his professional work. The change allows him to relax and easily fall asleep.

It hasn't been long since Lyall passed on, and at times my grief frightens me. It wasn't just losing Lyall that pulled me down, but the awful feeling that I would burden my family as long as I lived. Of course the feelings were mine alone. No one in the family gave me reason to think or feel this way. I realize now that these thoughts weren't rational.

Much to my surprise, I did not gradually emerge from this deep, black hole. I was snatched out of it suddenly.

I was invited by Focus on the Family to participate in a women's retreat in Palm Springs, California. In years past I had heard rave reviews from friends about the beauty of the desert and the sparkling, sunny climate. Lyall and I had thought it would be fun to plan a getaway in Palm Springs someday.

But now Poppa was gone, and I didn't want to go. Why would I want to spend four days with a bunch of gorgeous young women who were probably happily married? I'd drag them all down and, besides, I didn't want anyone to see me this depressed.

I'm grateful for the people God placed in my life during those very dark months. The elders in my church said to me, "Jean, you are no longer the iron lady. You must allow us to help you when you need it." My daughters said in no uncertain terms, "Mother, we insist you go to Palm Springs in spite of your feelings. A change of pace is what you need most right now." They made sure I got on that plane heading south.

There were women from across the nation at the retreat. Some of them I recognized as having been radio guests. Many of the women knew me from the years of broadcasting I had done with Dr. Dobson. During the first meeting we were asked to identify ourselves and say something meaningful about our lives. I suddenly found myself pouring out my heart and telling them that I was in desperate need of help. It was a very strange experience for me. I had thought I would "hide out" during the retreat and keep all my feelings to myself. It didn't turn out that way.

I soon discovered that many of the women had been reluctant to come to the retreat and felt guarded about their personal lives. It wasn't long before the others found themselves sharing their burdens, too. Vulnerability and transparency defined the time together.

Healing happened in my heart that week. The meetings were marvelous, and so were the fellowship and prayer times together. The cable-car trip to the top of the mountain, the breathtaking panoramic view below us, the delicious food, the fashion show of beautiful dresses that sparkled under the spotlights, the shining sun and warm desert air—all played an important part in my healing. It was a marvelous contrast to the sad events that had characterized my life during the previous two years.

My family will testify that after my oasis in the desert I never again fell back into that deep, black hole. I've learned lessons about reducing tension during the last couple of years that I didn't grasp when I was younger. Perhaps in the years ahead I will be able to look back and say that the years surrounding Lyall's death were filled with growth and maturity. For now I'm simply realizing that there are joys that come to us only through sorrow.

Deliberate Relaxation

During my clinical work I counseled people from all walks of life—the rich, the poor, the top executive, the person living on welfare. Through the years I've lost count of how many times I've heard, "I don't have time to relax."

Top executives struggle with high levels of frustration because too many people make too many demands on their time and abilities. Homemakers say the same thing. Even when they frantically work seven days a week, everything doesn't get accomplished. The work is *never* done!

Some take scheduled vacations, but their minds don't rest from work. Vacations are used to "get more done." Whether they're in a different country or a lovely exotic atmosphere, they're planning, phoning, scheduling, and programming. Time must not be wasted.

I've asked these driven executives and homemakers, "When do you take time off from work?" A variety of answers was given: "I love what I do." "My work [or my home] is my hobby." "It feels good to get things done and to have a day go as planned."

"But suppose everything doesn't go as planned?" I ask. "Then what?"

You see, there is an unattractive side to a driven life, and we create some of our own tensions. I have a hunch that the only way many of us can learn to relax is by purposely scheduling time away and putting our work on hold. Some of us can't trust ourselves to relax naturally because we feel guilty not being productive. Even when we obviously need to relax, it's difficult to stop interruptions. The tyranny of the urgent rules. How do I know? Because I'm a member of this club.

I have always enjoyed helping others, consequently my telephone constantly rings because of people in crisis. In earlier years I came home after long hours at the counseling center only to take more crisis calls at night. The person telephoning was usually desperate or suicidal.

Lyall always knew when it was one of "those" calls again. He frowned and made all kinds of signals, telling me to end the conversation. After I hung up, he would say, "Do you realize you were on the phone for over an hour? It's not fair to you or to us. You never get away from your work. We need to make some stringent rules about the telephone, for everyone's sake!"

Eventually I realized Lyall was right and learned to say, "No, I'm sorry, I cannot take your call tonight." Sometimes I referred the person to another therapist. Thanks to modern technology, I now have an answering machine that helps me set some limits.

I love to help. I never felt put-upon working sixteen-hour days. Now that I am older, I realize that lifestyle wasn't healthy for me or anyone, but someone would have had a hard time convincing me of this thirty years ago! Looking back, I realize I missed out on great opportunities for friendship. Heather, our youngest child, said, "You know what, Ma? Anyone would have to be mighty persistent to gain your friendship."

Her words were true. I was available when my friends were in trouble and needed a listening ear, but I wasn't a fair-weather friend. Rarely did I drop things and go places on the spur of the moment just for the fun. I know I'm not alone.

A survey on weekend leisure time commissioned by the Hilton Hotels Corporation confirms my suspicions. Many of us do not rest on our days off. Ninety percent of the workers in the survey reported returning to work exhausted after time off. Employers see the necessity of relaxation for their employees. Research shows a definite correlation between good self-care and work productivity. Some companies demand vacation time be taken within a twelve-month period of time. I know a number of church boards that insist their pastors take at least one day off each week in addition to an annual vacation. During this time they are not to indulge in any pastoral duties. They are to completely remove themselves and tend to personal and family needs.

I realize we live in a society that applauds workaholism, but in the long run, neglecting our personal lives isn't heroic.

It leads to burnout and wreaks havoc on our families and future. Dr. Peter Hanson, a specialist in stress management, says that most accidents occur on weekends, when people who are already tired cram more activities into their schedule. His point is that we need to fill our days off with rest and relaxation. He bluntly counsels his patients: "You *must* pamper yourself."[2]

Dr. Archibald Hart talks about the Scripture's teaching on the Sabbath. During biblical times, the Sabbath was spiritually, prophetically, and physically significant. One day out of seven was set aside for total rest. Everybody stopped work, even in the middle of the harvest, when time was a critical factor. Completely separating themselves from the mundane pressures of daily life, they focused on God and allowed Him to feed their souls. This was to prepare each individual mentally, physically, and spiritually for the coming week. Why this strict ritual? Because God created our bodies for times of hard work alternating with periods of relaxation. We weren't designed to operate in five-speed overdrive seven days a week.[3]

Do you want to reduce your tensions? Find time to stop and pull away from your responsibilities. Give your body and mind a chance to slow down. Even God rested after the sixth day of creation.

If we are naturally driven and achievement oriented, we will need to deliberately plan our moments of rest. It can be done. Do yourself a favor by scheduling buffer zones into your activity calendar.

Dehiscence

I had just arrived home from the airport. It had been hot while I was gone, so I rushed out to check my plants in the garden and greenhouse. *Good, the lovely maidenhair ferns survived*, I thought, examining the leaves closely. I was relieved. Christine, my granddaughter, had faithfully watered them.

Next I rushed over to my alpines to see the tiny bed of miniature wallflowers that had produced little seedpods. They were gone! Instead of plump, green, upright pods, there was nothing but withered, twisted bits of yellow straw. I bent down to take a closer look and noticed a few tiny yellow seeds still clinging to the twisted stems.

Without warning, a flashback took me to my childhood, where I stood with my botanist father in the garden. We were looking at fat little seedpods that had burst apart, sending their seeds far and wide. Father said, "How marvelous! Look, they have dehisced their seeds to scatter them. It took great heat for this to happen."

There seemed to be a lesson in this picture for me that afternoon. I went inside to my dictionary, curious to read the definition of *dehisce*. Webster's said, "to gape; the bursting open of a capsule, or a pod along a definable line, to discharge its contents."

Perhaps there are times when I can explode in a meaningful way, much like the little seedpods, I thought to myself, musing over the words in front of me. *Perhaps I can choose my own kind of explosions. I can dehisce, just like the plant, and this can serve as a functional outlet for pent-up emotion.*

I have recently discovered one way that I can purposely explode my feelings in the privacy of my own home, without harming anyone. I allow myself to sob from deep down in my soul. It's amazing the way this calms me. Research has shown that the hormones released during crying have a tranquilizing effect on our bodies. I think it is beautiful that our Creator made us with a built-in mechanism to reduce tension.

I've seen a good hard cry relieve tension in children, too. Laura, just on the verge of turning three, wanted to do something that wasn't permissible. She tried friendly persuasion, then some rather coy attempts to distract attention. Then she whined, and finally she burst into angry wails of protest against her mother, who refused to give in to her request. Suddenly, in the middle of her tantrum, she promptly stood up and said, "I'm going to my room to cry." A few moments later she shouted at the adults in the living room, "You be quiet—I'm crying!" This gave everyone a good laugh. Four or five minutes later the little girl came out of her room with her favorite doll in arm. That was it. We never heard another word about the incident. She acted as if it hadn't happened.

The fraternal twin to crying is laughter. I'm amazed by the stress-reducing benefits of a good, hearty laugh. A classic story illustrates my point.

James, a well-known business executive, died, and his family gathered together in his home prior to the memorial service. His five children had come a few days before his death, and the house was a flurry of activity. People from the church came and went, bringing food and flowers. The immediate family huddled together in the front room, talking and consoling one another. As visitors brought in deliveries, they were shocked to hear peals of hilarious laughter coming from the front room. The children were sharing funny memories of their father.

James was adored by his family, and his passing was a shocking blow. The children could not contain their grief. They mourned the loss of their beloved father and dreaded the public exposure at his funeral.

Carol, the mother of these five children, said many people were shocked at what might be interpreted as inappropriate behavior before a funeral, but she knew this was the only way they could relieve their grief before facing the ordeal of the funeral service. Laughter discharged their tension so they could cope with one of the most difficult hours of their lives.

Great heat for plants is like great tension for humans. The next time you're feeling overwhelmed with emotion, remember the lesson of the wallflower. Dehisce. Explode in a way that is productive. Let yourself cry or rock with laughter. It helps.

Dedicated Exercise

What are the first things to go haywire when we are stressed out? Healthy eating patterns, regular sleep, and exercise. It seems rather silly to talk about the importance of exercise, since so many books are written on the subject, but perhaps we'll all benefit from a brief reminder.

I cut out a few sentences from a magazine article recently to help me remember to stick to the basics. It said that exercise increases your fitness, helps your immune system, reduces stress, and lifts your mood.

Apparently good sleep patterns and exercise go hand in hand. Dr. Archibald Hart says, "People who exercise sleep better because it helps them use up surplus adrenaline, release muscular tension, ventilate the lungs, and create a physical fatigue that helps the onset of sleep."[4] He also says exercise lowers the risk of heart attack and elevates our moods. This is a tremendous bugger against burnout.

Unfortunately, in our frantic society, burnout is becoming increasingly common, and it is affecting both men and women. In the relevant book *Women's Burn Out*, the authors instruct those of us who are suffering burnout to move beyond the panic phase and take command of our bodies. They suggest hard aerobic exercise, saying, "Once you've got your body moving, your thoughts, attitudes, and feelings will experience a lift."[5] Their point is well made. Feelings follow actions. If we wait until we feel like exercising, most of us won't do it. We need to take charge of our bodies, and eventually positive moods will follow.

Science tells us why good moods follow. Research has documented the chemical hormone changes that occur in the brain when we participate in hard aerobic exercise. Endorphins, which act like natural mood elevators and tranquilizers, spill into the bloodstream, leaving us feeling less depressed and more calm. According to Dr. James Blumenthal, researcher at Duke University, there is also an increase of oxygen consumption during exercise, which does not occur during times of mental stress.[6] This probably explains why we hear people say "my head feels clear" after a vigorous workout.

One word of caution: the old rule, everything in moderation, applies to exercise, too. Overexercising can increase our stress. Running for pure pleasure has great stress-reducing benefits, but when an individual stops running for enjoyment and starts striving to compete, the exercise no longer serves to reduce tension.[7]

I well remember the strain of competing as a runner in intercollegiate sports in South Australia. As an eighteen-year-old, it was a grind, restricting my activities and going to bed every night promptly by 10:00 p.m. During competition I studied, ran, ate, and slept. There wasn't time for anything else. No doubt my stress spilled over to others around me.

Let me restate my point. Exercise is one way we can aggressively push stress out of our bodies, but if we tie exercise to competition, we'll likely lose some benefits. Many prominent national leaders recognize this and consistently exercise. Some insist that their employees do the same. Journalists go through all kinds of antics to capture pictures of the president running with his bodyguards and staff members.

For many years, Lyall and I were walkers. When the weather permitted, we walked outside, sometimes running for cover when rains caught us unexpectedly. Since the Northwest winters are cold and wet, we walked our two miles at the local mall. Poppa was always very focused, not letting the beautiful shop windows distract us.

Walking was a key to our good health, especially during the later years of our lives. The last decade brought many new and unique pressures. Walking helped clear our minds and ease the strains. I'm certain it enhanced Pa's keen mental abilities. During the week of his eightieth birthday, Lyall was invited to lecture students at Oxford University in England during their summer extension program. He didn't seem a day older than sixty to me. Aside from his conversion to Christianity, this was the greatest experience of his life.

Since Lyall's death I have occasionally walked out of sheer discipline to relieve the burden of grief. It has helped my moods and my health. He's not here to notice, but I can tell that those brisk walks leave me feeling a little less edgy. Even though sometimes it's a chore getting started, when I'm finished and the tennis shoes are peeled off, I know it was worth it, after all.

Deal with Unfinished Business

My lovely English garden now has large areas that are overgrown with weeds. It all started when Lyall became ill and wasn't able to tend to the grounds. Prior to his surgeries we put on our old grubby clothes and spent hours tackling those weeds together, but during his last couple of years, by necessity we spent our time doing quiet activities.

Every time I look out my kitchen window, I get angry. The weeds have bothered me for many weeks, and I can't seem to get away from that unsightly scene. Certainly this is unfinished business with a vengeance.

Common sense tells me, "Just tackle a little bit at a time, and then you'll feel better." The famous architect Frank Lloyd Wright taught his students to reduce their entire project down to its simplest parts. Yes, I do know how to tackle the garden, and soon I will give myself some time off to weed.

Unfinished business—most of us have it in our lives. A friend of mine once complained that her daughter had started seventeen projects without finishing any of them. Some of these projects were costly. "She says she feels defeated and inferior," the mother explained. "And now she's blaming her problems on living in the shadow of a high-achieving family. She's always keyed up. I feel uptight whenever I'm around her."

At the time my friend relayed this story to me, her daughter was seeing a psychiatrist. It was sad that this young woman failed to do what only she could do for herself. Nothing was going to change the achievers in her family. They would continue to work hard and reach goals. She needed to switch her focus from them and begin managing herself.

Unfinished business in relationships is fertile soil for tension. Not long ago I was asked to write an article for a family publication about children forgiving their parents. A long-forgotten incident came to my mind while I was working on that article. It happened between me and my mother during my adolescence.

For some reason Mother lashed out at me. She must have said something that hurt me deeply, because I resolved to never speak to her again. Extremely stubborn, I carried out my plan for days. One afternoon Mother came to me in tears, saying, "I beg your forgiveness. I never should have said those things to you. You did not deserve it, and I've felt badly ever since." Mother hugged me and cried.

While writing the article, I tried very hard to remember what Mother had said. I was curious to know what made a twelve-year-old retaliate in that way—but would you believe, I still cannot remember what she said.

I doubt I'll ever recall Mother's words, because when I heard her say, "I am sorry, please forgive me," the memory was blotted out. It was as though her harsh words were thrown out of my reach. The tension between us was dispelled as Mother and I dealt with our unfinished business. Neither of us shoved the incident aside, pretending it didn't happen. We addressed it. I'm thankful she initiated the conversation, because I don't think I would have at the time.

When we deal with unfinished business, anger and tension are discharged, and things can be put behind us. Of course, it isn't easy to say, "I'm sorry I hurt you. Will you please forgive me?" The natural human tendency is to say, "I had a perfect right to be angry and to speak my mind. I'd violate myself if I took back those words." Unfortunately, human tendencies don't always lead us to what we want. Any time we lash out and hurt others, we violate ourselves as well. We end up lonely, because people don't like to be with those who verbally slaughter them.

We are all human, and we are all going to make mistakes and say things that hurt others. That's a given. When we do, we need to address the hurt that has been done.

If we are Christian, we are going to feel unsettled until the matter is set straight. The Holy Spirit will constantly nudge us toward reconciliation. When we follow through, there is a good chance the memory will fade or at least lose its sting.

Recently, I had to deal with some unfinished business. A successful lawyer from New York was visiting her sister in Seattle. The women were twins and several times a year she flew out to be with her sister. It was a nice break from the extremely competitive life she led at the law firm in New York. Her last visit home had been six months ago, at which time she was ill, trying to recuperate. During her previous visit she seemed worried about her poor health and the hardship that was ahead of her when she returned to her job. I asked what she did for occasional relief from the pressures. Puzzled by my question, she said firmly, "There will be enough time for fun after I have finished my pressing cases."

I was concerned about her and gently tried to tell her that no one can be healthy if they work all the time. I suggested she deserved more fun than she was permitting herself. She left, and every now and then I prayed for her.

Then last month she visited her sister again. When I greeted her, I blurted out—in front of several other women— "You're the lady who does not know how to have fun. I hope such things have improved in your life."

She responded very quietly, "I think a lot depends on your definition of fun."

I told her that fun would be anything that relieved the tensions from her work. She was very quiet, and never said another word to me.

That night I worried about what I had said and was enraged with myself. I had been terribly brash. *This dear lady needed encouragement, love, and support,* I thought to myself, *not your rude, discourteous remarks!*

I couldn't get our conversation out of my mind. Each day that passed, the knot in my stomach tightened. I had to find her and make things right.

Fortunately I was able to arrange a meeting with her before the week was over. I asked her forgiveness. It was good for her to hear me say those words, but it was equally important for me. Oh, the relief that came from that time with her. She offered her forgiveness. That night when I laid my head on the pillow and closed my eyes, I knew the slate was clean. My offense was erased, and so was my tension.

Dare to Confront

At a three-day women's retreat I was asked to address the question, How can we deal with tension? Sue, a young friend of mine, was there, and she requested a few moments alone with me. We found a couple of chairs off in a private place, and her story unfolded.

"I have a gnawing problem with my sister-in-law. We used to be best friends, and now I don't want to see her anymore. It's awkward because I'm running out of excuses when my husband wants to invite them over.

"Joan and Bill view child rearing quite differently than we do. Frankly, their kids are a pain in the neck. When they come to our home, I try to manage the best I can, but believe me, it is a chore. I have to force myself to keep my mouth shut.

"Last week Joan told me we're ruining our kids by being too strict. She says I'm slavishly following my parents' outdated child-rearing methods and the etiquette training we do with the children is unnatural and ridiculous. But our children enjoy these times and have great fun acting out what *not* to do in certain situations."

"What do you think about what she said?" I asked.

229

"Jean, I don't agree with her. We listen to 'Focus on the Family' and follow the modern principles of child raising Dr. Dobson outlines. No one else thinks we are too strict. I resent her gossipy criticism. I think it irks her that the rest of the family praises our children and says nothing about her three spoiled brats. No one wants them around during family functions.

"The holiday season is approaching, and I don't know what to do."

She paused a moment, shifted in her seat, and continued.

"You have made me aware of my need to face my anger. This problem constantly hovers in the back of my mind. I can't get away from it. There are three family functions during the holidays. I suppose we could bow out altogether, but that wouldn't be fair to us. I don't want to miss being with the rest of the family just because they are there."

I agreed with Sue that something needed to be done, since things were progressively getting worse. Doing nothing was creating more tension. It seemed it would be worth the risk to confront her sister-in-law. Even if the confrontation didn't lead to the results she wanted, facing the source of her tensions could bring relief.

The thought of talking openly with Joan scared Sue. She typically avoided confrontation and was concerned her husband would blame her for causing trouble in the family. Not knowing how to confront, she asked me what to say.

All of us would agree that Sue was in a predicament. Things could go from bad to worse. She needed to approach it very carefully and prayerfully, knowing that the decision would affect the entire clan. I shared some thoughts with her.

"Perhaps you could phone your sister-in-law and ask her to meet you at a restaurant convenient for both of you. Neutral ground is the goal. Approach the subject by placing yourself on the hot seat. You could say something like, 'Joan, I am feeling very tense about something only you can understand. Maybe I am overreacting, but I think I'll feel better if I share my feelings with you. Several family members have told me that you are criticizing the way we are raising our children. You told me recently that you think we are too strict. Our children heard what you said from their cousins, and they feel put down.

"'Joan, I feel hurt, because our relationship is important to me. I want us to enjoy the friendship we had before this started. Ever since we became family, you have been my friend, and now I'm feeling bad about our friendship. Can you help me resolve my problem?'"

I went on to tell Sue that there were no guarantees the confrontation would have a happy ending. She couldn't predict the outcome or control Joan's response. I explained four possible outcomes that came to mind.

"Sue, there may be a nice ending to your story. Perhaps Joan will be touched by your openness and admit her wrong. She may be sorry for hurting you and agree to talk only to you when your ideas upset her. You never know. It's possible she may ask to hear your ideas on parenting.

"However, things could take a negative turn. She may accuse you of overreacting and say she has a right to voice her opinions. Or she could be indignant and deny she criticized you, saying you created the problem in your own mind. Or she may say others exaggerated her remarks to cause trouble, since she has different ideas about child rearing. She may be offended, abruptly walk out of the restaurant, and say the friendship is over. If she became your enemy, your husband's relationship with his brother would definitely be affected."

When the retreat ended, Sue went her way and I went mine. Some time later, at another women's meeting, she sought me out to tell me the end of the story. I remembered the situation well and was eager to hear the outcome.

"Oh, Jean, you won't believe what happened!" she exclaimed with glee. I could tell from the glow on her face that the news was good.

"After the retreat I went home and talked with my husband about Joan. I told him I wanted to risk talking honestly with Joan, even though there was no way to predict the results. I shared your warnings, and he was absolutely wonderful. He said he trusted my judgment and that my feelings meant more to him than anything else. His support meant so much to me.

"I followed your suggestions. I could not believe what happened. Joan broke down in tears, right there in the restaurant! She told me she resented our success with our children. Apparently the rest of the clan made no bones about telling her that they didn't like being around her kids. She wanted to come to us for help, but didn't want to admit her kids were out of control. She and her husband had talked about asking us how to make some changes as parents, but they just hadn't done it yet. Jean, she was genuinely sorry for upsetting me, and asked me to never give up on our friendship. She actually said she needed me."

Wow! That's the kind of story I love to hear. In all honesty, I would not have predicted that outcome. It seemed too good to be true. Nevertheless, Sue may never have gotten to that point of restoration had she not dared to confront.

Develop Empathy

They seemed like a nice couple who wanted advice about their children's quarreling. When I asked them to paint a picture of their home life, I was surprised with Mrs. Shaw's response. In a bland sort of way she said, "It's cluttered and not well kept. Dishes are piled on the counters and in the sink, and things are strewn across the floor in every room."

It seemed odd that she was so nonchalant about her disorderly home. Most women rationalize their messes, blaming it on the children or busy schedules. She did nothing of the sort.

Mr. Shaw agreed that his wife was a poor manager and also mentioned the dishes piled high in the kitchen. He also said he was raised by parents who were very neat and insisted he live by their high standards.

When I asked Mr. Shaw how he felt about his marriage, he said he was happy with his wife but hated the loud quarreling between their children. I was amazed at his acceptance of his wife's shortcomings. Sizing things up, I thought, *Here is a man who was raised by meticulous parents, and he's telling me his wife is a lousy housekeeper without a hint of anger.*

It didn't make sense. Other men I had seen in my office had very strong feelings about coming home to disorder. My research on 150 married couples confirmed this, too. Poor housekeeping was rated the number-one enemy of a happy marriage. For my own curiosity, I explored this further.

The next week, when Mr. Shaw talked with me alone, I said, "Mr. Shaw, I am puzzled about the way you described your wife's housekeeping, especially in light of your own upbringing. When your wife laughed about your parents' high standards and in the same breath called herself a slob, you laughed, too. It doesn't make sense that you aren't bothered by the difference in lifestyles."

I'll never forget his answer.

"Well, ma'am, you see, I understand her. If I had grown up like she did, I reckon I wouldn't do any better. She was raised in a pigsty and was never trained to be neat, like me. It isn't hard to make allowances for her when I think about

233

her childhood. I just try to pitch in and help her whenever I can. She'll probably get better in time. Besides, she has three children to look after, and the quarreling between the kids drains her."

I remember thinking, *Here is a beautiful example of empathy that allows a marriage to thrive.* Other couples might have said, "Our backgrounds are so different we will never make it," but Mr. Shaw chose to see things differently.

Do you see how empathy and low levels of anger are related? Empathy is the ability to recognize and appreciate the motivation of another, the ability to identify with another and at the same time to be different from him.[8] Empathy and sympathy are not the same. Sympathy is a feeling of compassion for another without an understanding of the motivation behind a particular action. Empathy includes both a feeling of compassion and an understanding of the motivation involved. When I empathize with someone, I actually take on the role of the other and interpret his behavior in the context of his experience, history, and background. This is how Mr. Shaw related to his wife. In so doing, his anger about their messy home was minimal.

Jane is another client who was empathic with her husband. The young couple lived in a little country home on a large piece of property, where snow fell heavily each winter. Two walkways outside needed daily shoveling so they could walk to and from their home.

Jane was a meticulous housekeeper. One afternoon she spent several hours polishing her tile floors while her husband was out tramping in the woods. As he plodded toward the front door in his big boots covered with mud and snow, Jane called from the kitchen, "John, don't come into the house with those muddy boots. Take them off outside. I just finished polishing the floor."

She had barely finished her sentence when John stormed into the kitchen, muddy boots and all, his face flushed with anger. In full voice he shouted, "Jane, don't you dare speak to me like that ever, ever again!"

Jane could not believe what she was hearing. She thought she had made a fairly ordinary request. John was usually fussy about keeping things clean, so his reaction caught her completely off guard. Why was he so insanely angry? As we talked together, she was able to answer that question for herself.

"When John was growing up, his mother was very capable, but dominant in a nice kind of way. Everyone knew she wore the pants in the family and made the important decisions. John was a quiet child and easy to raise, but during his teenage years he resented the way his mother controlled his life. She told her friends he was born to be a missionary and she planned to give him the best training possible. She told John that from the moment of his conception, she had dedicated him to God for mission work on the foreign field. John never said anything, but decided on his own to study business at a large secular university. This was a complete surprise and tremendous disappointment for his mother."

Jane saw the picture. During childhood, John stuffed his feelings and never talked back to his parents. As an adult he still harbored well-covered anger toward his controlling mother. When he heard the words, "Don't come in the house with your muddy boots on," he didn't hear Jane. He heard his mother issuing commands.

Jane's empathy allowed her to remain calm about the incident. She realized his outburst wasn't directed at her, and she separated herself from his anger. She was the trigger, not the cause. Because of her empathy the conflict was short-lived. After a while, John's rage died down and they talked about what happened between them.

As I reflect on nearly forty years of clinical work, I notice some similarities among people who are chronically tense. Rarely do they listen to anyone but themselves. They tend to be impatient, not wanting to take time to be fully informed about how others see things. They jump in and finish sentences, then make wrong conclusions because they don't listen with all their faculties. Always trying to juggle three or four things at a time, they can rarely focus on the single issue at hand. Their distracted mind shuts down chances for developing empathy. Unfortunately, tense people live in a constant state of anger because they do not understand why others say what they say or do what they do.

Empathy can douse fires and calm stormy relationships. When we understand the why behind someone's reaction, the original negative stimulus that produced the tension can be canceled. This happened to me some years ago.

I saw an older lady in our church standing alone by the doorway. I had seen her before, but couldn't remember her name. I had not been attending the church long and was still trying to sort out who was who. I walked over to her and said, "I don't think I know you. I wanted to come introduce myself."

She peered sharply at me and retorted, "Of course you know full well who I am. You are very insulting!"

I felt awful! I walked away thinking she was a very ill-tempered woman whose remark was totally out of line. I decided to avoid her in the future.

Later I asked someone else who she was, and then talked with her daughter-in-law about the incident. I am so glad I did. She helped me see the pain behind her outburst.

"Oh, Mrs. Lush, if you knew the story of her life, you would understand. Her husband was a prominent leader in the church, and she lived in his shadow. When they were raising their young family, she spent night after night at home alone with the children, while he went to church for one activity or another. She was left out of everything. He is retired now and very healthy and active. Her health is poor, so nothing has changed.

"She made tremendous sacrifices for her family without any recognition, especially from him. Years ago she tragically lost her son and hasn't been the same since. So when you approached her and said you didn't know her, her life script was being played out once again. You see, she remembered that you had spoken to her husband on a number of occasions, yet you never noticed her."

That conversation changed my attitude in less than five minutes. Understanding her pain made it difficult for me to be angry. The next week, instead of avoiding her, I went out of my way to be friendly. When I saw her at church I apologized for not recognizing her the Sunday before. I said, "Jane, I am so sorry about what I said last week. I could have kicked myself afterward. Of course I know who you are. I've heard folks in the church talk about your excellent Bible teaching. Sometimes I get confused because this church is so big and there are so many people." That was the beginning of a dialogue that continued until she died.

Researchers who specialize in the study of human nature say that empathy is psychogenic, meaning it is apparent to a great degree in certain personalities from birth. The ability to be empathetic may be partly determined by inheritance. However, researchers also say that it is possible for anyone to develop empathy.[9]

I agree with their conclusions. I have even seen people who are naturally self-absorbed and insensitive learn empathy. It is possible, and most of us have room for improvement in this area.

If we want to develop empathy, we must examine our listening skills. It takes effort and determination to listen well. It's much easier to jump into a conversation with advice or to jabber about our own experiences. Heart specialist Dr. Redford Williams says it well: "When you break in on someone during a conversation, it sends the message that your ideas are more important than what they are saying. Learn to listen. Force yourself to keep your mouth shut until they have finished. An attentive posture will also send the message to the other person—I value you and your ideas."[10]

The prerequisites for empathy are a closed mouth and open ears. As you listen, try to use all your faculties. Study not only the words that are said, but also the tone of voice and body language of the one who is talking. Try to step into their shoes and understand their world. Your empathy will be a gift to others and a dependable way to reduce your own tensions. Simply put, "Be quick to listen, slow to speak and slow to become angry" (James 1:19). The payoff will be worth it.

Dig for Blessings

Recently I received a telephone call from Oklahoma. An old friend identified herself and said, "I just received news that your Lyall died last spring. It has been exactly ten years since my husband was killed. I have just one thing to share with you: you will know God as you have never known Him before."

While trying to control a sudden flow of tears, I said, "Yes, Evelyn. I know."

Even during my most despondent moments, I sense God's love for me. In the dark hours before dawn I plead for God's strength to uphold me each day. All of my natural self-control and stoicism has failed. Until now, I could control my tears. Even when my beloved first grandson died of cancer at age seven, I remained dry-eyed while disintegrating inside. For years I hardened my feelings toward little boys who crossed my path.

Things are different now. I cry daily, wondering if life will ever be joyful again, yet I am keenly aware that God is with me. In time, I'll see His blessings.

I believe many of life's greatest blessings come wrapped in struggle paper. Unwrapping those blessings takes time. It's a process consisting of several phases.

In the first stage we panic. Life delivers an unexpected package to our door, and we don't like what we find inside. Shock, anger, confusion, and grief set in. A terrible sense of desperation lurks. We wonder, "Will I survive this pain? Has God deserted me?"

Then comes the endurance phase. A chronic state of tension leaves us feeling overwhelmed. We want to rise above the emotional tides, but something keeps pulling us back under. Every now and then we catch a gulp of air and the waters still, but soon the waves and wind kick up and we plunge to the depths again. "Doesn't God know I've had enough? I can't take any more." In this phase we simply cope.

Finally, we enter the renewal phase—recovery, restoration, re-creation, refreshment, growth—the healing of our soul, the heightening of our powers. We sense the blessings.

Those who have gone before us knew these blessings. George Mueller, a man of tremendous faith, founded some of the world's most famous orphanages in England. His name will live forever. When one of his admirers asked him how he developed such great faith, he said, "The only way to learn great faith is to endure great trials. I have learned faith by standing firm amid testings."

Another great figure of faith who has influenced my life was Madame Guyon of France. During a privileged and happy childhood, she was honored for her intelligence and beauty in King Louis the Fourteenth's court. As the custom of the day demanded, Madame Guyon's parents arranged for her to marry. The man chosen was twenty years her senior. Unable to feel love for him, she wrote in her memoirs, "I was no sooner at home with my husband than I saw clearly that it would be to me a house of sorrow."

Madame Guyon's wealthy mother-in-law lived with the newlyweds and ruled the household. Her husband meekly submitted to his mother's dominating ways and persecuted his new wife. They refused to allow Madame Guyon to raise her own children because of her faith in Christ. She was cast aside as the family heretic.

In the later years of life, Madame Guyon was finally freed from the tyranny of this family. Traveling throughout France, she taught about God's love in highly sophisticated circles. This woman became an aristocrat of the seventeenth century and played an important role in French history.

In my deepest moments of despair, I despise the pain of this world. It makes me angry. It drains my energy and will to live. I'm learning, though, that if I dig deep enough, good can always be found. Somewhere there are golden blessings to be uncovered.

The psalmist talks about digging up blessings in the deserts of life: "Happy are those who are strong in the Lord, who want above all else to follow your steps. When they walk through the Valley of Weeping it will become a place of springs where pools of blessing and refreshment collect after rains! They will grow constantly in strength" (Ps. 84:5–7 TLB).

The Valley of Weeping was a dry, dreary place without natural rains. When pilgrims traveled through this valley, they dug down through the parched soil to find an underlying source of water. The new springs became a blessing for the weary travelers and all those who later followed their path.

We all have times when life leads us into arid wastelands. The scenery is void of color and beauty. High heat and winds make life unbearable. We huff and puff and strain and toil. But in the midst of our desert storms there is a source of blessing. What Jesus promised the woman at the well, He promises you and me: "Whoever takes a drink of the water that I will give him shall never, no never, be thirsty any more. But the water that I will give him shall become a spring of water welling up continually within him unto eternal life" (John 4:14 AMP). Not only does He want to quench our thirst, He also wants to transform our dry, cracked lands into conduits through which rivers of His healing power can be released to water other barren, thirsty souls. Now that's the kind of blessing I love to receive.

19

Don't Look Back

It's 5:30 a.m. Outside my window I can see wispy clouds blanketing the trees. This was one of Lyall's favorite times of day. He used to bounce out of bed and rush to the garden to watch the mists move in and out of the giant fir trees surrounding our home. "Jean, you must join me for this spectacular sight!" he would command. Together we would watch the sun climb lazily over the greenery, shedding its brilliance through hovering mists. Several times during his terminal illness I heard him say, "My best painting is still ahead of me. I'm going to paint a picture of our English cottage garden, like Monet." He was always looking forward.

Lyall had a knack for keeping his sights in front and not looking back. He didn't like dwelling on the past, unless the memories were of happy times. Oh, he had as good a reason as any to carry grudges from days gone by. He had known severe injustice. Some of these painful times were a result of his childlike trust in people. In spite of his genius, he used poor judgment in some business endeavors, and the costs were extreme.

No matter what happened, Lyall never held a grudge. He refused to allow failures and disappointments to drag him down. He was always the first to say, "It's time to let go and let God take over." I believe this is what kept Lyall light-hearted and smiling. He chose to look on the positive side of life. One evening we received news that we had suffered a tremendous financial setback. The first thing he said was, "Well, there is one thing in my life that is a great success. My marriage."

It was nice being married to a man who didn't look back. I wish more of this quality had rubbed off on me. Looking back has been something I have fought most of my life. I'm sure I'm not the only one who has heard barred doors slam shut behind them. Life has a way of leading us into prisons: poor health, siblings who outperform us, unloving parents, a marriage that didn't turn out as we expected, sick babies. We've all been locked in at one time or another.

Paul knew about prison firsthand, although I'm sure the experience came as quite a surprise. God had asked him to deliver a message to the Gentile nations. Paul had a great sense of adventure and was eager to take the message of God's love to the ends of the earth. With unconquerable zeal, he set out on his travels, but militant Jews who opposed his efforts threw him in prison. History tells us he was locked in a dungeon for two years, chained to Roman guards around the clock.

One day free, the next, incarcerated. Paul had no idea chains would be a part of God's plan. Sore feet, maybe, but not chains.

It's funny how those chains played a major role in accomplishing God's plan. While Paul was in prison, people from far and wide visited him. They brought him gifts money couldn't buy—open ears and hungry hearts. When the prison gates closed behind them, these visitors carried Paul's message throughout the entire Roman Empire, as far west as Gaul and Spain.

Visitors weren't the only ones who helped Paul facilitate God's plan. The Praetorian guards to whom he was chained played a key part, too. Historians tell us there were nine divisions of one thousand men that served as Praetorian guards. At all times one of these companies was in the palace.

The divisions were constantly rotated from one assignment to the next. Some guarded political prisoners like Paul, while others protected the Emperor in the palace. Some divisions were sent by special orders to the far borders of the empire. The short rotations prevented soldiers from developing personal relationships that interfered with their duties.

The guards worked six-hour shifts. Each day four shifts of soldiers locked and unlocked themselves from Paul's chains. New companies came each week. This means that Paul had four different guards each day who were a "captive audience." That's 28 people a week, 112 guards a month, over 1,300 soldiers a year. In two years, a lot of folks heard the message of God's love! This doesn't even include the visitors who carried Paul's message outside the prison walls.

Long before his imprisonment, Paul wrote a letter to the courageous new Christians in Rome, encouraging them in their faith. This letter, known today as the book of Romans, is recorded in the New Testament. Paul told the Romans he longed to visit them, to spur them on in their spiritual growth. In later years his longing was fulfilled, but it took an imprisonment.

During the two years Paul was in that cold, dark dungeon, he penned a letter to the church of Philippi. In his opening paragraphs he said,

> I want you to know this, dear brothers: Everything that has happened to me here has been a great boost in getting out the Good News concerning Christ. For everyone around here, including all the soldiers over at the barracks, knows that I am in chains simply because I am a Christian. And because of my imprisonment many of the Christians here seem to have lost their fear of chains! Somehow my patience has encouraged them and they have become more and more bold in telling others about Christ.
>
> Philippians 1:12–14 TLB

No "Poor me." No pity parties. He kept looking forward.

He says, "I keep on forgetting the things which are behind. I keep on reaching for the things ahead. I keep on pressing toward the mark."[1] It was a futuristic perspective, a daily choice, an hourly choice.

I've learned that I live in a chronic state of tension when I cling to the past and blame myself and others for what was and is. Looking back, there is one thing I would do differently: I would not waste so much energy struggling against what I couldn't change. So many times I rebelled when I should have yielded. Others rarely saw this, but I knew my heart.

Paul tells us this life is like a race—an ironic analogy coming from a man who was limited to a few small steps a day. We cannot run our race if we're weighted down by the past. My anger over my losses was like a millstone around my neck. It slowed me to a standstill, particularly as I grew older. It was only through yielding and looking ahead that the ropes on which those millstones hung were severed. Finally I was free. How I wish I had made these choices years earlier.

Instead of failure, Paul's prison experience became God's gateway to his success. God's purposes were fulfilled in those confining cells; confinement sponsored refinement. It's a paradox, isn't it? Out of the crucible of suffering and constraint came the greatest achievements Paul ever accomplished.

I have a hunch Paul knew his message reached far beyond his cell. I'll bet he heard that people in the uttermost parts of the empire were buzzing with the news of Christ. I'll bet when he died in Rome, a city he had never seen, he and the Lord smiled. Mission accomplished, calling fulfilled, race won, even with those rusty old chains around his ankles.

That's God. He's not intimidated or limited by our prison walls. We might be, but He's not. He marches right into the prison cells of life and says, "Even in the confines of this dreary dungeon, my plan for your life will go forward. There's no looking back. I will accomplish my good work in you."

I have a destiny. So do you. Let's allow Lyall and Paul to rub off on us. Put the past to rest; look forward; dream big dreams; go for the gold. Run to win, even when chains are clanking along behind you.

Notes

Chapter 1

1. "Too Much Stress Burns Out Brain Cells," *Everett Herald*, May 7, 1990, 1.

2. *Webster's Third International Dictionary*, vol. 3 (Chicago: William Benton, 1966), 2260.

3. *Webster's New Collegiate Dictionary* (Springfield, MA: Merriam-Webster, 1956), 838.

4. Redford Williams, *The Trusting Heart: Great News about Type A Behavior* (New York: Random House, 1989), 76.

5. Cited in Archibald D. Hart, *Adrenalin and Stress* (Dallas: Word Publishing, 1988), 29–30.

Chapter 2

1. Hart, *Adrenalin and Stress*, 213.

2. S. I. McMillen, *None of These Diseases* (Grand Rapids: Revell, 1979), 97.

3. Spurgeon O. English and Stuart M. Finch, *Introduction to Psychiatry* (New York: W. W. Norton and Co., 1957), 21.

4. Otto Fenichel, *The Psychoanalytic Theory of Neurosis* (New York: W. W. Norton and Co., 1945), 391, 512.

5. English and Finch, *Introduction to Psychiatry*, 19.

Chapter 3

1. Frank B. Minirth and Paul D. Meier, *Happiness Is a Choice* (Grand Rapids: Baker Books, 1978), 150.
2. Quoted by Alexandra Stoddard in, "Seven Steps to Self-Esteem," *McCall's* (May 1991), 144.

Chapter 4

1. Sandra Aldrich, interview, January 1992.
2. Pam Vredevelt, *Empty Arms: Emotional Support for Those Who Have Suffered Miscarriage or Stillbirth* (Eugene, OR: Multnomah Press, 1984), 9, 19, 23, 122–24.
3. Aldrich, op. cit.
4. Neta Jackson, interview, January 1992.
5. Liz Gill, "Why Crying Is Good for the Soul," *New Ideas* (March 1990), 42.

Chapter 6

1. Michelle Morris, "What Causes Stress, What Does Not," *McCall's* (March 1991), 74.

Chapter 8

1. Material on pages 89–93 is from Jean Lush, *Mothers and Sons: Raising Boys to Be Men* (Grand Rapids: Revell, 1988), 126–28, 130–31.
2. Louise Bates Ames, *He Hit Me First* (New York: Red Dembner Enterprises, 1982), 18.
3. Lush, *Mothers and Sons*, 46–48.
4. Margaret Mack, interview, January 1992.

Chapter 9

1. S. L. Israel, *Diagnosis and Treatment of Menstrual Disorders and Sterility* (New York: Paul S. Hoeber, 1959), 176.
2. Material on pages 106–114 is taken from Jean Lush, *Emotional Phases of a Woman's Life* (Grand Rapids: Revell, 1987), 155–63.
3. Michael O'Hara and Jane Engeldinger, "Postpartum Mood Disorders: Detection and Prevention," *The Female Patient, Practical Ob/Gyn Medicine* 14 (June 1989), 6.
4. Dr. David Lush, interview, January 1992.
5. O'Hara and Engeldinger, "Postpartum Mood Disorders," 23.

6. Larraine Dennersteen and Eylard Van Hill, *Psychosomatic Gynecology* (Park Ridge, NJ: The Parthenon Publishing Group, Ltd., 1986), 139.

7. Ibid., 145.

8. Ibid., 140.

9. Penny Wise Budoff, *No More Menstrual Cramps and Other Good News* (New York: G. P. Putnam's Sons, Penguin Books, 1981), 137–38.

10. Katharina Dalton, *Once a Month* (Claremont, CA: Hunter House, 1987), 28.

Chapter 10

1. Helene Deutsch, *The Psychology of Women: A Psycho-analytic Interpretation*, vol. 1 (New York: Grune and Stratton, 1944), 214.

2. Ibid., 456, 459, 461.

3. Therese Benedek, *Studies in Psycho-somatic Medicine: Psychosexual Functions in Women* (New York: Ronald Press, 1952), 368–69, 371.

4. Paula Weideger, *Menstruation and Menopause* (New York: Alfred A. Knopf, 1976), 209.

5. Frank J. McGowan, *Because You Are a Woman* (Greenwich, CT: Fawcett Publications, Inc., 1962), 59.

6. Penny Wise Budoff, *No More Hot Flashes* (New York: Warner Books, G. P. Putnam's Sons, 1983), 3.

7. Material on pages 128–35 is from Jean Lush, *Emotional Phases of a Woman's Life* (Grand Rapids: Revell, 1987), 182–90.

8. Joe S. McIlhaney Jr., with Susan Nethery, *1250 Health-Care Questions Women Ask* (Grand Rapids: Baker Books, 1985), 76.

9. Katharina Dalton, *Once a Month* (Claremont, CA: Hunter House, 1987), 154.

10. Ibid.

11. Ibid., 155.

12. Penny Wise Budoff, *No More Menstrual Cramps and Other Good News* (New York: G. P. Putnam's Sons, Penguin Books, 1981), 193.

13. Dalton, *Once a Month*, 144–48.

14. Weideger, *Menstruation and Menopause*, 61.

15. The following section, pages 136–39 is from Lush, *Emotional Phases*, 191–203.

16. McIlhaney, *1250 Health-Care Questions*, 183.

Chapter 11

1. Alfred Ells, *One-Way Relationships* (Nashville: Thomas Nelson Publishers, 1990), 79–80.

Chapter 13

1. Theodore Isaac Rubin, *The Angry Book* (New York: Macmillan Publishing Co., 1969), 137.

2. Dwight L. Carlson, *Overcoming Hurts and Anger* (Eugene, OR: Harvest House Publishers, 1981), 87.

3. Harriet Lerner, *The Dance of Anger* (New York: Harper & Row, 1985), 32.

Chapter 15

1. Shirley Chisholm, *The Good Fight* (New York: Harper & Row, 1973), 32.

2. Barnard, Bryn Mawr, Goucher, and Radcliffe colleges, "One Hundred Women of the Century," *Good Housekeeping* (July 1985), 261–68.

3. Frank B. Minirth and Paul D. Meier, *Happiness Is a Choice* (Grand Rapids: Baker Books, 1978), 175.

Chapter 16

1. Gloria Vanderbilt, *Woman to Woman* (New York: Doubleday and Co., 1979), 190.

2. Alexandra Stoddard, "Putting Your Life in Order," *McCall's* (September 1989), 140.

Chapter 17

1. Redford Williams, *The Trusting Heart: Great News about Type A Behavior* (New York: Random House, 1989), 81, 16, 19.

2. Archibald D. Hart, *Adrenalin and Stress* (Dallas: Word Publishing, 1988), 167–68.

3. Lillian B. Rubin, *Just Friends: The Role of Friendship in our Lives* (New York: Harper and Row, 1985), 61.

4. Ibid.

Chapter 18

1. John Stuart Mill, Mary Jane Moffet, and Charlotte Painter, eds., *Diaries of Women* (New York: Random House, 1974), 403.

2. George Hirsch, "How Running Relieves Stress," *The Runner* (August 1986), 41.

3. Archibald D. Hart, *Adrenalin and Stress* (Dallas: Word Publishing, 1988), 51.

4. Ibid., 100, 161.

5. Herbert J. Freudenberger and Gail North, *Women's Burn Out* (New York: Penguin Books, 1986), 177.

6. Dr. James Blumenthal, quoted in Hirsch, "How Running Relieves Stress," 41.

7. Ibid.

8. Ernest W. Burgess and Paul Wallen, *Engagement and Marriage* (Chicago: J. B. Lippincott Co., 1953), 624–39.

9. Ibid., 635, 639.

10. Williams, *The Trusting Heart*, 189.

Chapter 19

1. John F. Walvoord, *Philippians—Triumph in Christ* (Chicago: Moody Press, 1971), 92.

Family therapist **Jean Lush** was well known for her radio and television outreach and as the author of the bestselling *Emotional Phases of a Woman's Life*. Jean Lush passed away near her home in Edmonds, Washington.

Pam Vredevelt is a bestselling author, popular conference speaker, and licensed professional counselor at NW Counseling Services in Gresham, Oregon.

Raise your boys
to be their best!

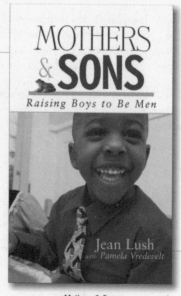

Mothers & Sons

Revell
a division of Baker Publishing Group
www.RevellBooks.com
Available wherever books are sold.